PUBLIC HEALTH ENGINEERING

AUTHOR

Dr. Rinku Kumar

Lecturer, Department of Civil Engineering, Government Polytechnic Mankeda,
Agra, Uttar Pradesh, India

REVIEWER

Mr. Ajay Vikram Ahirwar

Associate Professor,
Department of Civil Engineering, National Institute of Technology Raipur, Amanaka, Chhattisgarh, India

KHANNA BOOK PUBLISHING CO. (P) Ltd.
4C/4344, Ansari Road, Darya Ganj,
New Delhi, India

All India Council for Technical Education
Nelson Mandela Marg, Vasant Kunj,
New Delhi, India

Dear Readers,

To prevent the piracy, this book is secured with HIGH SECURITY HOLOGRAM on the front title cover. In case you don't find the hologram on the front cover title, please write us to at contact@khannabooks.com or whatsapp us at +91-99109 09320 and avail special gift voucher for yourself.

Specimen of Hologram on front Cover title:

Moreover, there is a SPECIAL DISCOUNT COUPON for you with EVERY HOLOGRAM.

How to avail this SPECIAL DISCOUNT:

Step 1: Scratch the hologram

Step 2: Under the scratch area, your "coupon code" is available

Step 3: Logon to www.khannabooks.com

Step 4: Use your "coupon code" in the shopping cart and get your copy at a special discount

Step 5: Enjoy your reading!

ISBN: 978-93-5538-870-4

Book Code: DIP502EN

Public Health Engineering

by Dr. Rinku Kumar

First Edition: 2026

Originally Published by:

All India Council for Technical Education, Ministry of Education, GOI

Exclusively Published & Distributed by:

Khanna Book Publishing Co. (P) Ltd.

4C/4344, Ansari Road, Daryaganj,
New Delhi (INDIA)

Visit us at: **www.khannabooks.com**

Write us at: **contact@khannabooks.com**

To view complete list of books,
Please scan the QR Code:

KPH

Printed in Bharat.

प्रो. टी. जी. सीताराम
अध्यक्ष
Prof. T. G. Sitharam
Chairman

सत्यमेव जयते

आज़ादी का अमृत महोत्सव

अखिल भारतीय तकनीकी शिक्षा परिषद्
(भारत सरकार का एक सांविधिक निकाय)
(शिक्षा मंत्रालय, भारत सरकार)
नेल्सन मंडेला मार्ग, वसंत कुंज, नई दिल्ली–110070
दूरभाष : 011–26131498
ई–मेल : chairman@aicte-india.org

ALL INDIA COUNCIL FOR TECHNICAL EDUCATION
(A STATUTORY BODY OF THE GOVT. OF INDIA)
(Ministry of Education, Govt. of India)
Nelson Mandela Marg, Vasant Kunj, New Delhi-110070
Phone : 011-26131498
E-mail : chairman@aicte-india.org

FOREWORD

Engineers are the backbone of any modern society. They are the ones responsible for the marvels as well as the improved quality of life across the world. Engineers have driven humanity towards greater heights in a more evolved and unprecedented manner.

The All India Council for Technical Education (AICTE), have spared no efforts towards the strengthening of the technical education in the country. AICTE is always committed towards promoting quality Technical Education to make India a modern developed nation emphasizing on the overall welfare of mankind.

An array of initiatives has been taken by AICTE in last decade which have been accelerated now by the National Education Policy (NEP) 2020. The implementation of NEP under the visionary leadership of Hon'ble Prime Minister of India envisages the provision for education in regional languages to all, thereby ensuring that every graduate becomes competent enough and is in a position to contribute towards the national growth and development through innovation & entrepreneurship.

One of the spheres where AICTE had been relentlessly working since past couple of years is providing high quality original technical contents at Under Graduate & Diploma level prepared and translated by eminent educators in various Indian languages to its aspirants. For students pursuing 2nd year of their Engineering education, AICTE has identified 87 books, which shall be translated into 12 Indian languages - Hindi, Tamil, Gujarati, Odia, Bengali, Kannada, Urdu, Punjabi, Telugu, Marathi, Assamese & Malayalam. In addition to the English medium, books in different Indian Languages are going to support the students to understand the concepts in their respective mother tongue.

On behalf of AICTE, I express sincere gratitude to all distinguished authors, reviewers and translators from the renowned institutions of high repute for their admirable contribution in a record span of time.

AICTE is confident that these outcomes based original contents shall help aspirants to master the subject with comprehension and greater ease.

(Prof. T. G. Sitharam)

DEDICATION

This book is dedicated to my son, Riyansh, the sunshine of my life and I hope that this book will inspire him in the future as he inspire me to write.

ACKNOWLEDGMENT

I am grateful to the authorities of AICTE, particularly Prof. T. G. Sitharam, Chairman; Dr. Abhay Jere, Vice-Chairman; Prof. Rajive Kumar, Member-Secretary and Dr. Sunil Luthra, Director and Reena Sharma, Hindi Officer Training and Learning Bureau for their planning to publish the books on Public Health Engineering. I sincerely acknowledge the valuable contributions of the reviewer of the book Mr. Ajay Vikram Ahriwar, Associate Professor, Department of Civil Engineering, NIT Raipur for his contribution in the form of his vast knowledge and experience on the subject.

I want to express my deepest gratitude to my **parents Mr. Chhidda Lal and Mrs. Kashmiri Devi** for their belief in me. Their unwavering support is the foundation for all my endeavours.

To my wife, Mrs. Sandhya Singh, your patience and understanding makes every achievement sweeter for me. Your continuous support and encouragement make every challenge easy for me.

To my beloved son, Riyansh Singh, you are the light of our life. Your smile and curiosity about every small and big thing inspire me to work hard. Your laughter and imagination are always a source of motivation for me.

I would like to offer special thanks to Mr. Anil Kumar, Dr. Poonam Kumari, Mr. Dharmendra Singh, Mr. Vishwanath Pratap Singh, Dr. Sandeep Panchal, Dr. Sudhanshu Singh, Mr. Shri Krishna and Mr. Ashok Siddharth to provide moral support, encouragement and helped us in every possible way.

This book is an outcome of various suggestions of AICTE members, experts, and authors who shared their opinions and thoughts to further develop engineering education in our country. Acknowledgments are due to the contributors and different workers in this field whose published books, review articles, papers, photographs, footnotes, references, and other valuable information enriched me at the time of writing the book.

Dr. Rinku kumar

PREFACE

The subject "Public Health Engineering" is one of the most important subjects in civil engineering. A thorough understanding of water and wastewater treatment is an asset for civil engineering students and practicing engineers. Accurate estimates of water demands help the stakeholders in making the right decisions on the construction and development project of a town. The budget allocation by the government departments for the different water projects is also based on population forecasting. The students who have good knowledge of water and wastewater treatment can choose their career as Environmental Engineers. Keeping in mind the purpose of wide coverage as well as to provide essential supplementary information, the topics recommended by AICTE are included in a very systematic and orderly manner throughout the book. Efforts have been made to explain the fundamental concepts of the subject in the simplest possible way.

During the process of preparation of the manuscript, different standard textbooks from the National and International publishers are referred. As the subject is based on the practical aspect of civil engineering, the realistic problems are discussed in detail with solved numerical examples. The book covers all types of details of sources, demand, quality and quantity of water required for diploma-level students.

The unsolved questions included in this book are designed to make the students think about the problem. It will help in boosting the problem-solving skills of the students. The students will find it interesting to read this book. The information presented in this will enhance the curiosity among the students and will develop their interest in public health engineering. The provisions of Indian Standard Codes, discharge limits, and recent test for determining quantity of water are discussed in detail which will help professional engineers in updating their knowledge on the subject. The book is prepared to build a strong foundation of knowledge on the subject of public health engineering. The presented book will prepare engineering students to apply their knowledge of water and wastewater treatment to solve the problems in planning and management of developing a new town projects.

I sincerely hope that the book will inspire civil engineering students and professionals to learn and discuss the concepts and ideas of the subject of public health engineering. Further suggestions and comments are welcome for the improvement of the book for its upcoming editions. It is my pleasure to place this book in the hands of the teachers, students, and civil engineering professionals. Working on different aspects covered in the book was a big pleasure.

Dr. Rinku kumar

OUTCOME BASED EDUCATION

For the implementation of an outcome-based education, the first requirement is to develop an outcome- based curriculum and incorporate an outcome-based assessment in the education system. By going through outcome-based assessments evaluators will be able to evaluate whether the students have achieved the outlined standard, specific, and measurable outcomes. With the proper incorporation of outcome-based education, there will be a definite commitment to achieve a minimum standard for all learners without giving up at any level. At the end of the program running with the aid of outcome-based education, a student will be able to arrive at the following outcomes:

PO-1: Engineering knowledge: Apply the knowledge of mathematics, science, engineering fundamentals, and an engineering specialization to the solution of complex engineering problems.

PO-2: Problem analysis: Identify, formulate, review research literature, and analyze complex engineering problems reaching substantiated conclusions using first principles of mathematics, natural sciences, and engineering sciences.

PO-3: Design / development of solutions: Design solutions for complex engineering problems and design system components or processes that meet the specified needs with appropriate consideration for the public health and safety, and the cultural, societal, and environmental considerations.

PO-4: Conduct investigations of complex problems: Use research-based knowledge and research methods including design of experiments, analysis and interpretation of data, and synthesis of the information to provide valid conclusions.

PO-5: Modern tool usage: Create, select, and apply appropriate techniques, resources, and modern engineering and IT tools including prediction and modeling to complex engineering activities with an understanding of the limitations.

PO-6: The engineer and society: Apply reasoning informed by the contextual knowledge to assess societal, health, safety, legal and cultural issues and the consequent responsibilities relevant to the professional engineering practice.

PO-7: Environment and sustainability: Understand the impact of professional engineering solutions in societal and environmental contexts, and demonstrate the knowledge of, and need for sustainable development.

COURSE OUTCOMES

After completing this course, students will be able to:

CO-1: Know the procedure to identify the sources of surface and subsurface water.

CO-2: Estimate the quantity of drinking water required for a population.

CO-3: Draw labelled layout for water supply scheme.

CO-4: Device suitable water treatment technique.

CO-5: Evaluate the characteristics and suggest treatment of sewage.

Course Outcomes	Expected Mapping with Programme Outcomes *(1- Weak Correlation; 2- Medium correlation; 3- Strong Correlation)*						
	PO-1	PO-2	PO-3	PO-4	PO-5	PO-6	PO-7
CO-1	3	2	2	1	1	2	-
CO-2	3	3	3	2	2	3	1
CO-3	3	3	3	2	2	3	2
CO-4	3	2	2	1	3	2	2
CO-5	3	3	3	2	2	3	-

ABBREVIATIONS AND SYMBOLS

List of Abbreviations

General Terms			
Abbreviations	**Full form**	**Abbreviations**	**Full form**
lpcd	liters per capita per day	CPCB	Central Pollution Control Board
ppm	Parts per million	BOD	Bio-chemical Oxygen Demand
IS	Indian Standards	COD	Chemical Oxygen Demand
MPN	Most Probable Number	MOHUA	Ministry of Housing and Urban Affairs
GOI	Government of India		
DC RPM	Direct Current Round Per Minute	MOEFCC	Ministry of Environment, Forest and Climate Change

List of Units and Symbols

Symbols/ Units	Description	Symbols/ Units	Description
m	Metre	%	Percentage
G	Specific density of particle	km	Kilometer
T	Temperature	C	Celcius
d	Diameter of the particles	KN	Kilo Newton
cm	Centimetre	g	Gram
mg	Milligram	sec	second
Kg	Kilogram	min	minute
l	liter	hr	hour
ml	Milliliter	m^3	Cubic meter
m^2	Square metre	cm^2	Square centimeter
mm	millimeter	$l/hr/m^2$	Liter per hour per square meter
°	degree	Cm/sec	Centimetre per second
g	gram	μm	Micrometre

GUIDELINES FOR TEACHERS

To implement Outcome Based Education (OBE) knowledge level and skill set of the students should be enhanced. Teachers should take a major responsibility for the proper implementation of OBE. Some of the responsibilities (not limited to) for the teachers in OBE system may be as follows:

- Within reasonable constraint, they should manoeuvre time to the best advantage of all students.
- They should assess the students only upon certain defined criterion without considering any other potential ineligibility to discriminate them.
- They should try to grow the learning abilities of the students to a certain level before they leave the institute.
- They should try to ensure that all the students are equipped with the quality knowledge as well as competence after they finish their education.
- They should always encourage the students to develop their ultimate performance capabilities.
- They should facilitate and encourage group work and team work to consolidate newer approach.
- They should follow Blooms taxonomy in every part of the assessment.

Bloom's Taxonomy

Level	Teacher should Check	Student should be able to	Possible Mode of Assessment
Create	Students ability to create	Design or Create	Mini project
Evaluate	Students ability to justify	Argue or Defend	Assignment
Analyse	Students ability to distinguish	Differentiate or Distinguish	Project/Lab Methodology
Apply	Students ability to use information	Operate or Demonstrate	Technical Presentation/ Demonstration
Understand	Students ability to explain the ideas	Explain or Classify	Presentation/Seminar
Remember	Students ability to recall (or remember)	Define or Recall	Quiz

GUIDELINES FOR STUDENTS

Students should take equal responsibility for implementing the OBE. Some of the responsibilities (not limited to) for the students in OBE system are as follows:

- Students should be well aware of each UO before the start of a unit in every course.
- Students should be well aware of each CO before the start of the course.
- Students should be well aware of each PO before the start of the program.
- Students should think critically and reasonably with proper reflection and action.
- Learning of the students should be connected and integrated with practical and real-life consequences.
- Students should be well aware of their competency at every level of OBE.

LIST OF FIGURES

LIST OF TABLES

CONTENTS

1 Sources, Demand and Quality of Water

UNIT SPECIFICS

Through this unit we have discussed the following aspects:

- *To understand various sources of raw water for the water supply scheme*
- *Different types of intake structure*
- *Different methods for population forecasting*
- *Overview of quality of water*
- *Physical, chemical, and biological characteristics of water*
- *Understand the demand of water in a town or city*

To help the students in the visualization of the content and to enhance their practical knowledge, the figures are provided in 2D. The content in this unit offers practical knowledge and will help thc students in decision-making during the fieldwork.

This unit contains short and long answer-type questions along with multiple choice questions, a list of references, and suggested reading so that one can go through them for practice. Some QR codes are given which can be scanned for more information on various topics of interest and to get extra knowledge.

RATIONALE

This unit on sources, demand, and quality of water helps the students to develop an idea about the various sources of raw water and the design and layout of the intake structure. It explains the objectives and components of the water supply scheme. The various water sources used for the water supply are discussed. A brief discussion of various types of intake structures is done. The various water demands are also discussed and the method of population forecast is well explained. The different physical, chemical, and biological parameters are discussed. The content covered in this unit is important to understanding sources, demand, and quality of water for water supply schemes.

The knowledge of various sources of water and their quality is essential for civil engineering students. The students can apply the knowledge of the sources and demand during designing water treatment plants. The knowledge gained in this unit will help the students to identify suitable sources for different types of demand for water supply scheme. The students can apply their knowledge in the selection and implementation of desired quality of water during the treatment process. The concepts in this unit will help the student in effective supervision of working water treatment plants.

PRE-REQUISITES

A basic knowledge of water properties is required.

UNIT OUTCOMES

The list of outcomes of this unit is as follows:

U1-O1: *To learn the sources of the water supply scheme*

U1-O2: *To understand the various demand*

U1-O3: *To learn the method of population forecasting*

U1-O4: *To determine the quality of water*

U1-O5: *To propose a suitable source, demand and quality for water treatment plant*

Unit-1 Outcomes	EXPECTED MAPPING WITH COURSE OUTCOMES (1- Weak Correlation; 2- Medium correlation; 3- Strong Correlation)				
	CO-1	CO-2	CO-3	CO-4	CO-5
U1-O1	3	1	-	-	-
U1-O2	2	1	-	-	-
U1-O3	-	2	-	-	-
U1-O4	-	3	-	1	-
U1-O5	-	2	2	-	-

1.1 INTRODUCTION

Resources such as air, water, and food are very critical for the survival of human beings. These resources are so important, if they are polluted they can cause harmful diseases such as respiratory problems caused by air pollution similarly water-borne diseases (diarrhea, cholera, hepatitis, etc.) can be caused by water contamination and food poisoning can be caused by food contamination. As we can see the resources which are essential for life can become the reason for harmful for human being when they get contaminated. A probe can be written related to this "Human beings can survive without love but they cannot live without water". Three forms of water are present on Earth i.e. liquid form, solid form (snow), and gaseous form. All these forms combined help in providing luxuries and comfort in life, in addition to its basic function to human beings. Human beings become helpless, if there no water in there house or in tap. Apart from human beings water is also required by plants, animals and other living beings.

In history, we can see that civilizations and mankind only developed or settled near the bedside of rivers or lakes. In those times water is only required for domestic use. In that era water was carried out from a well with the help of animals and people took that water to their houses by lifting the vessels on their heads. For purification of water, Sushruta Samhita (an ancient Indian literature) describes that & quote; it is good to keep the water in the copper vessels and put a piece of Charcoal in it. As we get more civilized they demand for water continues to grow as water is required for some other use. In today's era, apart from domestic use water is required in industries, manufacturing companies, public use, fire-fighting, and sewerage systems. Now, the means of transporting the water has been changed and water is supplied in a closed pipeline to every household. These modern water supply schemes are designed in such a way as to cater to the demands of the increasing population and transport the water free from any contamination. Therefore, to ensure a good quality and quantity water supply, it becomes imperative to plan and design water supply schemes. Well-defined knowledge is therefore required to arrange a modern water supply scheme. As the supply of water and water contamination is related to human beings health. Therefore, in these books, we will study how a water supply scheme should be and what quality and quantity of water we have to supply to meet various demands of the modern era.

1.1.1 OBJECTIVES OF WATER SUPPLY SCHEME

The various objectives of the water supply scheme are mentioned below

- To provide safe portable/drinking water to people in their required quantity (135 lpcd) and quality (as per Indian standard codes)
- To make water easily reachable to the consumer with the desired pressure in the supply pipeline.
- It should be planned in such a way as to meet the needs of future demand increase due to an increase in population
- There should be provision for adequate water supply in case of emergency uses such as fire- fighting demand or festivals
- To make the distribution system economical and reliable for the community
- To collect the wastewater generated from the community and treat before its disposal.
- To plan the mitigation measures of the water pollution through the policy making.

1.1.2 COMPONENTS OF A WATER SUPPLY SCHEME

The various components of a water supply scheme in the municipality of town/city are:

a. **Water supply sources:** These are different sources such as river, lakes, ponds and ground from where we get the raw water for supply to the town if it is clean and free from pollution or else it will be sent to the treatment units.

b. **Different Treatment Units:** In this process, water is made free of different impurities (physical, chemical, and biological). Physical impurities are removed by screening and a primary sedimentation tank. Chemical impurities are removed by coagulation/flocculation and biological impurities are removed with the help of filtration and disinfection.

c. **Storage Tanks:** In these units, the treated water is stored before distribution to the households. Different types of storage tanks can be made based of the availability of land and topography. Different types of storage tanks are Ground storage tanks, overhead storage tanks, and underground storage tanks.

d. **Water distribution network:** It helps in providing the treated water with sufficient pressure to the households. It consists of different sizes and lengths of pipes and pump houses.

1.2 SOURCES OF WATER

The different suitable sources for different types of demand for water supply scheme can be broadly classified into two categories:

1. Surface water
2. Sub-surface water

1.2.1 SURFACE WATER

In these different sources of water comes under from which we can directly get water on the surface of earth. Those surface water sources are:

- Lakes and Natural ponds
- Rivers
- Reservoirs

1.2.1.1 LAKES AND NATURAL PONDS

These are natural depressions on the surface of the earth, which get filled with water and are known as natural ponds or lakes. Both of these terms are interchangeable depending on the size of the depression, if the size is comparatively very large it is known as a lake otherwise it can be said as a pond. Water in these ponds or lakes is contributed by surface run-off from rainfall. The quantity of water in lakes or ponds depends on the catchment area which is generally small in size and annual rainfall of that area. As the water in these lakes and ponds is smaller in quantity they are not used as main sources of water supply in the large towns., but in cases where no other alternatives are present then these lakes can be used as primary source of supply for example in Mumbai different lakes are used for water supply. The quality of water from lakes and ponds are generally good and they do not require much of treatment.

1.2.1.2 RIVERS

Different streams and springs merge to form a river. Rivers as the source of supply of water is used from ancient civilizations as most of the ancient towns and cities are situated on the bank of river. Rivers are mainly of two types:

- Perennial river
- Non-Perennial river

Perennial rivers are those rivers which contains water throughout year due to rainfall water during monsoon season and in summer due to melting of snow. They can be used as the primary source of water supply in a city. Non-perennial rivers are also known as seasonal rivers as water is only present during monsoon season. They can only be used for water supply when the water is stored during monsoon season by making dams.

The water quality of river is not good and reliable as it's contains a lot of impurities in the form of silt, sand and suspended particles. Completely or partially treated wastewater is discharge into the upstream of river which make it somewhat suspected for contamination. Therefore if river water is used for a water supply scheme it should be purified before supply to the public.

1.2.1.3 RESERVOIRS

When there is a low flow of water in the river it becomes difficult to supply desired quantity or during monsoon when there is a high flow due to flood the water supply from the river become difficult to operate. An artificial structure known as a dam or reservoir is created to store the water for supply. The quality of water stored upstream of reservoirs is the same as that of lakes. The water store can also be used for other purposes such as irrigation. A reservoir consists of a structure that can hold a large quality of water, a gate to discharge extra water, and different values to regulate the flow of water.

Reservoir design is a vast topic in itself and not discussed but some important feature of a reservoir is given below:

a) Selection of the location of the dam.
   - It should be such that local availability of material near the site.
   - The foundation of the natural bed should be strong enough to bear a large amount of weight without undergoing settlement
   - Catchment area
   - Water quantity and quality
   - Site easy to accessible

b) Capacity to store the water
   - Average monthly rainfall data to determine
   - Run-off coefficient
   - Topography and contouring of the site to be carried out

c) Different types of dams
   - Earth dams
   - Rockfill dam
   - Arch dam

d) Different losses of water from reservoirs

- Losses due to evaporation
- Losses due to absorption
- Losses due to percolation

1.2.2 SUB-SURFACE WATER

Sub-surface water is also known as underground water. This type of water is stored in an underground reservoir due to infiltration. The quality of this water is very good as it gets naturally filtration as water passes through soil pores. This water is sometimes rich in dissolved salt, minerals, and different gases. The extent of these minerals and salts depends on the minerals ore from which water has been passed during its movements to reach the underground water table. There is very little chance of getting this water contaminated by bacteria.

The underground water is generally brought to the surface by artificially construction such as tube wells, infiltration galleries, or by natural processes such as springs. Underground water availability at a place depends on two important properties of soil. They are

- ➢ Porosity
- ➢ Permeability

Permeability is defined as the ability of the soil sediment to allow or pass water within the soil sediment. It means the more permeable the soil has greater the tendency to pass water through itself. Sandy soil has higher permeability than clayey soil as it has coarse particle size which has more pores to pass the water as compared to finer particle size.

Porosity is defined as the ratio of the volume of pores or voids in the soil to its total volume. It is expressed in the percentage. If the percentage is high it means the soil has high porosity. Sandy soil has higher porosity as compared to other types of soil. In water supply scheme the aquifer which contains sandy soil is more preferred as compared to other type of aquifers.

Different sources of underground water are:

1. **Spring:** Springs is that part of the earth's surface from where underground water naturally flows on the surface. These springs sometimes occur due to water filling in the aquifer during raining season at the point that its water table increases and coincides with the surface they are known as intermittent springs. The water quality of spring water is good as it is pure and can be directly used for domestic purpose without much of treatment.
2. **Wells:** Rainwater infiltrating into the soil during surface run-off gets trapped beneath the impermeable layer and taken out by making pot or drilling on the ground, which is known as well. In India, a large population depends on wells for water supply. The porosity of the soil plays a major role in identifying the amount of water present in the well. If there is higher porosity, the aquifer will easily collect more quantity of water. The wells are of different types:

a) **Shallow wells:** These wells are not deep, the tap the water from the upper permeable layer i.e. known as the water table. In summer, when there is a drop-down in the water table due to excess demand this type of wells dries up or the quantity of water decreases. Generally shallow well's diameter varies from 2 m to 6 m and its depth is around 3 m to 10 m. They have a low discharge rate of 180 to 300 liters per minute. Water obtain from shallow well has better quality then surface water but required certain treatment before distribution. Figure 1.1 shows the configuration of the shallow well.

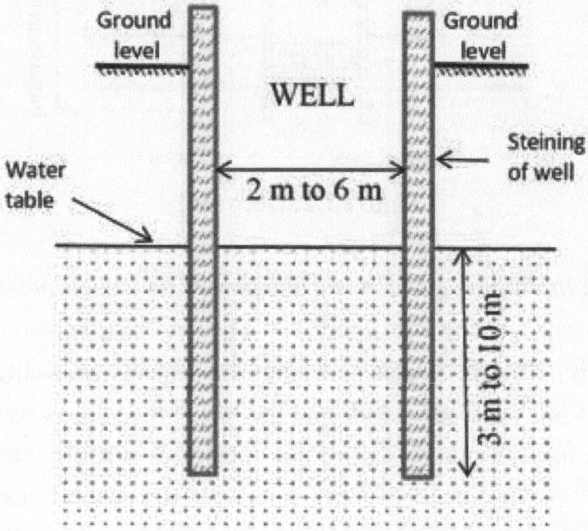

Figure 1.1: Shallow well

b) **Deep Well:** Deep well as name suggested they are having a very high depth as they penetrate many layers of permeable and impermeable aquifers as shown in figure 1.2. The quality of water obtained from deep wells is very clean and pure as impurities from the surface get trapped on the top impermeable layers. Sometimes water contains some minerals and saline in nature due to presence of mineral ores in the permeable layer. Sometimes, it requires certain treatment before the distribution of water to the community. The water from the deep well travels to the permeable outcrop to the site. Outcrop is the site where the aquifer is exposed to the surface of earth. Strainers (figure 1.2) are provided to the face of the pipe which is located in the permeable layer. This strainer has small holes through which water moves from the aquifer to the well. A tube well is an example of a deep well.

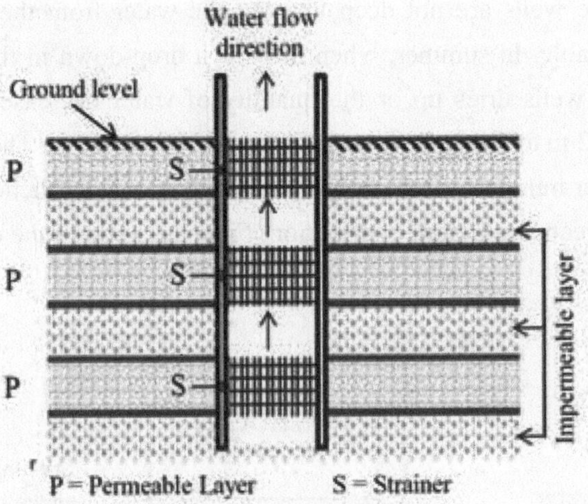

Figure 1.2: Deep well

c) **Infiltration Gallery:** *Infiltration galleries are like horizontal tunnels present near the river bank and* pass through water strata as shown in figure 1.3. They are also known as horizontal wells. These gallery's water quality is much cleaner and purer than open-type wells. The infiltration gallery's walls are made up of brick masonry work and the top of the well is covered with RCC. Water in galleries is collected through porous drain pipes located at suitable intervals in aquifer along the length. Porous drain pipes are often covered with gravel and pebbles to stop the entry of fine sand. These galleries are laid along the slope of water and water from these galleries is sent to sump and from there to further treatment and distribution. These are generally constructed at a depth of 3 to 5 m below ground level.

d) **Infiltration Wells:** Infiltration wells are also used to collect underground water near the banks of river by making small wells in series at shallow depths (3 m to 6 m). They collect river water from the open bottom end. Walls of infiltration wells are made up of brick masonry and the top of the well is covered as shown in Figure 1.4a. A manhole is provided at the top for inspection of the well. Different infiltrations well as shown in figure 4b are connected to one jack well by porous drain pipe and from there water is uplifted and sent for treatment and distribution to the community.

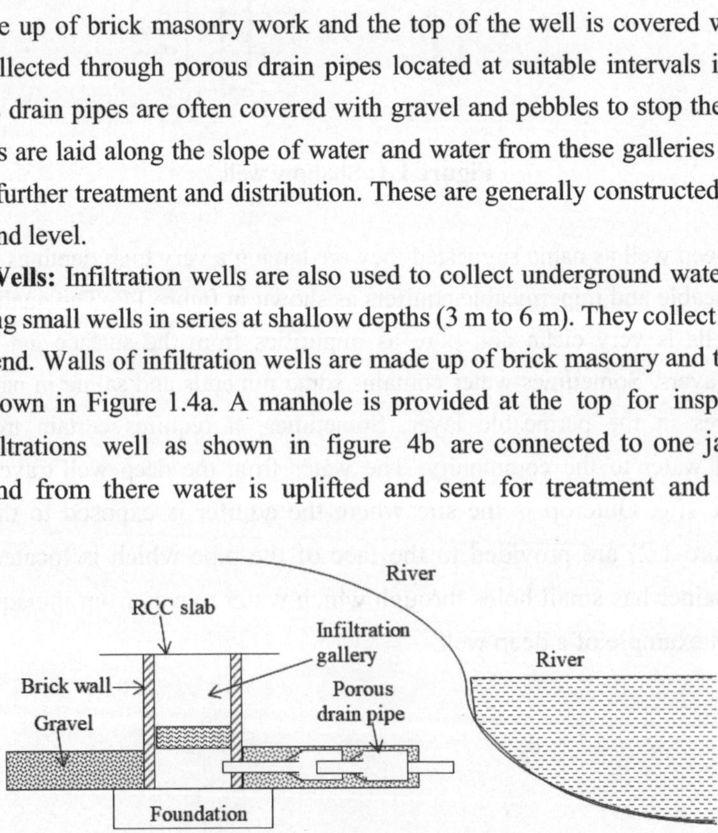

Figure 1.3: Infiltration Gallery

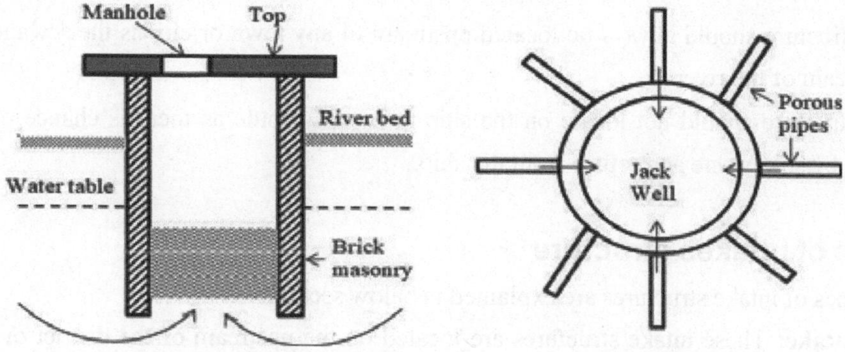

a. Section of infiltration well b. Jack well

Figure 1.4: Infiltration well

1.2.3 INTAKE

Intakes are the structure that is built on the shore of the surface water source such as rivers, lakes or ponds to get water out for treatment and distribution to the community. In places where the surface water source (rivers, lakes, ponds) lies at a higher altitude then gravity flow is possible to supply water to the treatment units but in the case where rivers flow at lower altitudes then the intake structure also contains water pumps to supply water to the treatment units.

The intake structure should be firm enough to protect itself from the high current of flowing river and raging waves. These are constructed at the start of water supply pipes, therefore protecting them from damage by debris, snow, etc. This intake structure can be small in size to support conduits for water supply or sometimes they are larger to cater to the pump, screen, motors, and living quarters for operational personnel.

1.2.4 Factors governing the location of an intake structure

The following points to be considered while selecting the suitable location for different types of intake structures for water supply to a particular town or a city:

- The location of the intake structure should be near the treatment units to reduce the cost of water distribution to the city.
- The location of the intake structure in the river should be such that it gets good quality water out from the source so that the cost of treatment can be reduced
- Site location should be such that the necessary water quantity available during the year
- The structure's location should be such that it can meet the water requirement of future demand.
- Location should be easily accessible during floods and do not get submerged during floods.
- When there is a meandering river, the intake structure should be avoided near sharp turning but in case they have to be located, the intake structure should be located on a concave bank in place of the convex bank.

- Intake structure should always be located upstream of any town or city as the sewage gets disposed downstream of the river.
- Intake structure should not locate on the ship navigation route as there is chance of water getting polluted by ship waste and refuse from the ship.

1.2.5 Types of intakes structure

The various types of intake structures are explained in below section:

1) **River Intake:** These intake structures are located on the upstream of the district or a town having straight water flows and should have a minimum flow throughout the year. Location points should have a minimum pollution. These intake structures are made near the banks of the river or inside the river having sufficient depth to meet the water requirement in the summer season. If the flow is low during the summer season wears are constructed to meet the demand. These intake structures are doubled wall circular in shape made of masonry or concrete having a diameter of 3m to 5m. Motors and pumps are placed in the upper section of the well. This section is known as the pump house and remains dry. While lower section contains screens and suction pipes and remains wet as shown in figure 1.5.

Pumping is required in this type of intake to lift the water as the river flows below the ground level. Pen stocks are installed at various vertical holes in the collector wells. Penstock pipes contain screens on the mouth of the opening to protect the well from impurities such as weeds, wood, water creatures, etc. The various vertical holes help in maintain the water throughout the year in the summer seasons.

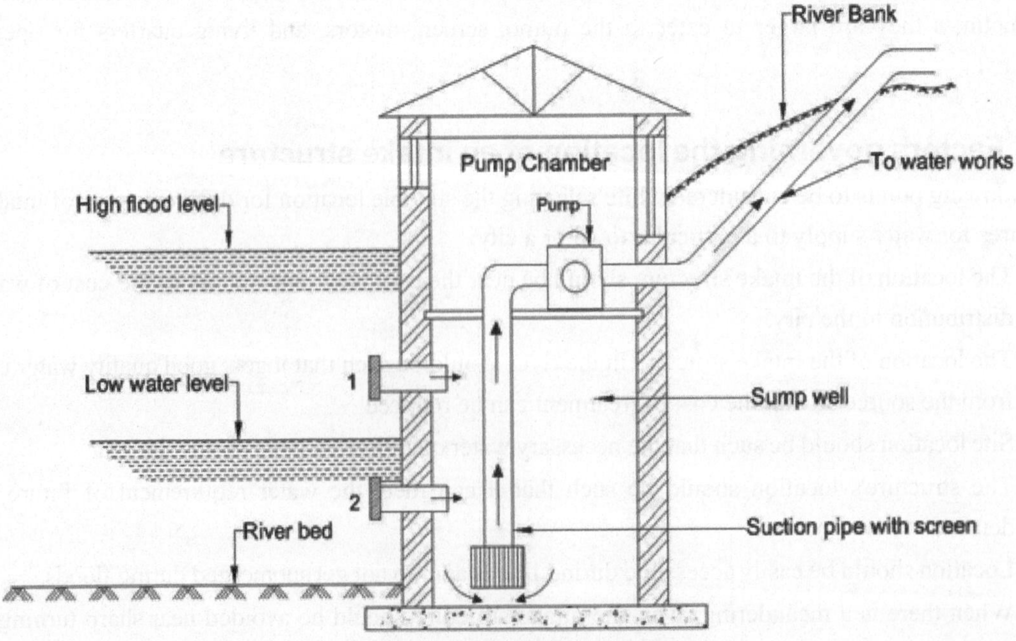

Figure 1.5: River intake

2) Canal Intake: These types of intake structures are made when there are no alternate source of water is present for drinking purpose. Water is taken from an irrigation canal. Generally, irrigation canals are located above the ground level so there is no need for a pumping station. The water reaches the water works through gravitational flow. A circular chamber of masonry works or concrete is made inside the canal to form canal intake as shown in figure 1.6. The canal intake structure is covered with a concrete slab from the top. A hole is made on the wall of concrete from where the water enters into the intake structure. The mouth of the hole is covered with iron screens to protect it from entering of impurities into the intake structure. Inside the chamber, a bell-shaped inlet pipe covered with mesh is installed from where the water is transported to the waterworks. For controlling the flow of water in the outlet pipe a sluice valve is placed which can be opened and closed from the roof of the chamber.

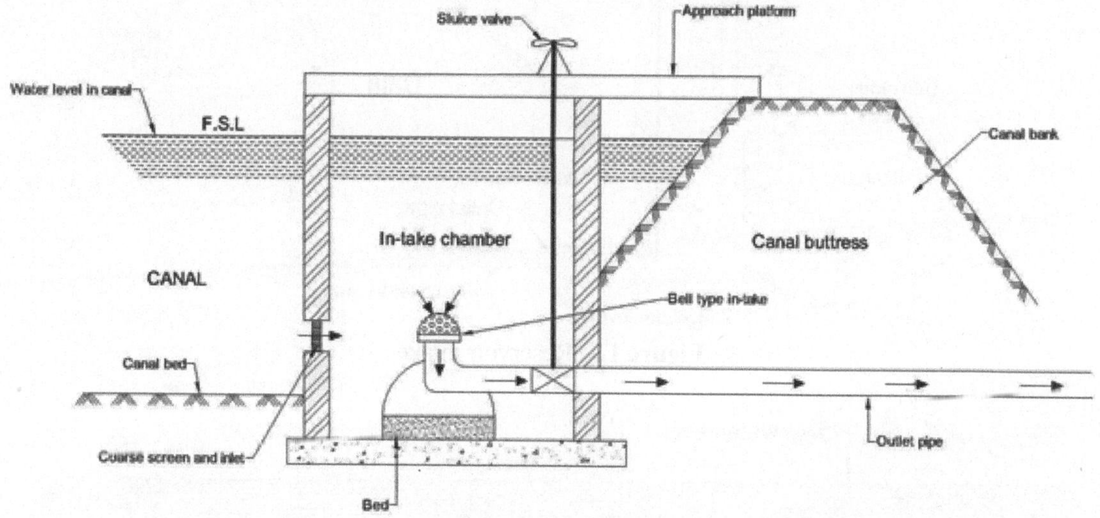

Figure 1.6: Canal intake

3) Reservoir intake: These structures are made in the dam to take water from the reservoir. There are several inlets pipe connected to circular chamber which is made of concrete or masonry works at various vertical height as shown in figure 1.7. These inlet pipe openings are covered with mesh wire know as screens to protect from various floating impurities in the reservoir. The purpose of installing different inlet pipes at different vertical heights so that water availability remains equal during a drop in the water level. A sluice valve is attached inside the inlet pipes to control the water flow. It can be opened and closed from the top of the tower. Water in the reservoir has higher level than the ground level, so the water flow automatically due to gravitational flow. Foot bridge are made from the dam to the top of the reservoir intake to reach the intake well for inspection and operation and repair works. The wall of the intake structure should be firm enough to protect it from the continuous strike of water waves and floating ice blocks.

4) Lake intake: Lake intake is the structure constructed to take water from the lakes and streams. Structures are made at the bottom of the lakes as generally water in the lakes gets dropped during summer seasons. These intake structures are also known as submerged intake. Submerged structure sides are protected with the help of boulders and the top is covered with concrete slabs as shown in figure 1.8. The intake chamber is covered with a thick wire mesh lid for the flow of water and to protect the chamber from entering impurities. Water enters into bell shaped mouth chamber through mesh. Exhaust pipes are connected to the bottom of the chamber to transport water from the chamber to the water works site. If the depth of the lake is very high the exhaust pipes are connected to the sump well and from there the water is transported with the help of a pump to the waterworks site.

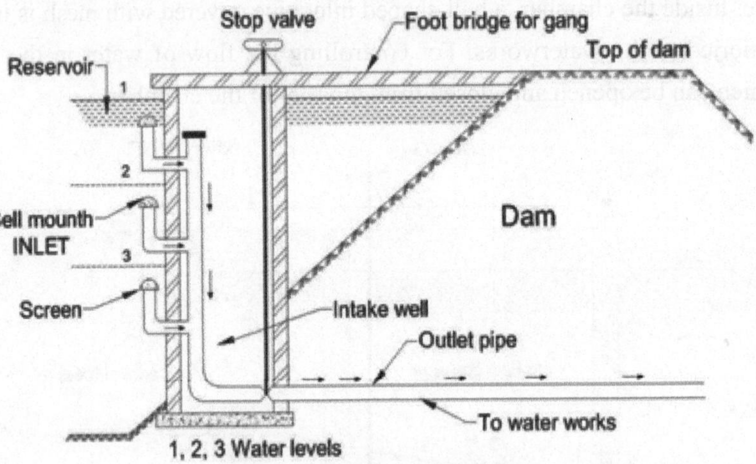

Figure 1.7: Reservoir intake

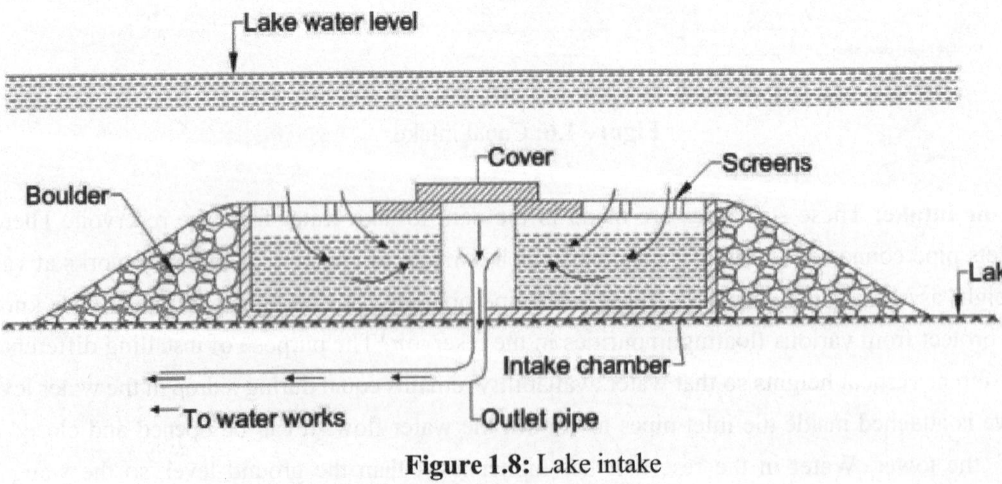

Figure 1.8: Lake intake

1.3 Demand of water

Demand of water play an important role in planning and design of water supply scheme. The demand of water for a person for his daily needs 24 hour a day is known as per capita per day consumption of water. Demand in generally evaluated in liters per capita per day (lpcd). According to Indian standard code 1172-

1993 (reaffirmed 2007) the daily demand of normal consumption for per person having a population of more than 1 lakh with a flushing system is 150-200 lpcd, but it gets reduced to 135 lpcd for lower income group and economically weaker section of society these values depends on the prevailing conditions.

1.3.1 Factors affecting rate of demand

The water demand varies from one place to another place. The demand of water is also not same for per person per day for all state. The various factors which affect the rate of demand are given below:

- **Climate:** Climate condition such as hotter places or colder places has a direct impact on the consumption of water. In winter season the water demand is less while in summer season demand increase as more water is required for bathing and other domestic activity such as washing. air cooling and sprinkling in lawns and gardens. In extreme weather conditions where the temperature remains in negative temperature the water requirement is more as there water tap remains open continuously to avoid the freezing of pipes.
- **City population:** In bigger city they have larger population as compared to smaller cities or towns so the large cities have higher lpcd compare to smaller cities. In larger cities the demand of water is more due to clean environment as there is sewerage system for flushing which required for water. Larger cities also have more business activities and larger commercial and industrial area which increase the demand of water. The average water demand of Indian cities based on per capita demand for different populations is shown in Table 1.1.

Table 1.1: Water demand based on population

S. No.	Size of population	Water demand in lpcd
1	0 – 20,000	Less than 110 liters
2	20,001 – 50,000	110 to 150 liters
3	50,001 – 2,00,000	150 to 240 liters
4	2,00,001 – 5,00,000	240 to 275 liters
5	5,00,001 – 10,00,000	275 to 335 liters
6	More than 10,00,000	More than 335 liters

- **Types of people and their habits**: Higher-class people who are richer consume more water due to their high living standards. Middle-class people consume average water demand while lower-class or slum people require less water. Economic conditions directly affect the water demand for a particular town.
- **Water Quality:** Water quality is playing an important role in water demand for a particular area. If water quality is of a higher standard more the water demand of that area as more population demands of water supply as compared to private wells and hand pumps. Public uses higher standard

water supplies for various daily activities as compared to water have unpleasant odour and taste. Industries also used this water for their boiler feed which required higher standard water which in turn increases the water demand.

- **Water supply system:** Supply of water in a town or community occurred either by supplying water in the peak demand hours of morning and evening or there will be a continuously supply of water for 24 hours in a day. In the periodic water supply, there is a lower demand for water as compared to continuously supply because in periodic supply there is lesser loss of water and consumers use the water more carefully in convenient and saving mode. But in some case the intermittent supply not save much of water as compared to continuous supply. In these cases where person store water in larger cans for future uses but thrown away this water when there is fresh water available in the tab.
- **Sewerage facilities:** In a town or a city where the sewerage system is developed the people use large amount of water in flushing system which in turn increase the per capita per person water demand.
- **Pressure in the distribution pipes:** When there is proper pressure in the distribution system water can easily reach to the upper 3rd and 4th story, which allows person to use water more freely. These in turn increase the water demand. Other factors such as losses and water leakage will also increase as the pressure increases in the water distribution system, which leads to an increase in water demand.
- **Method of water charging:** Water charging is generally done by two methods in a town. They are:

  I. By flat rate system

  II. By meter reading basis

In the flat rate system, the water charge is fixed for a month and its do not depend on the amount of water used. In these methods, the waste of water is more as people not used in careful manner and the water demand is high. In metering system there is a water meter installed at the head of the water connection of an individual house. The person only used that amount of water which is necessary as he/she has to paid amount on the basic of consumption.

- **Water for Industrial and commercial use:** Due to presence of large industries and commercial hubs in a town increases the water demand of that particular area. Large industries require an adequate amount of water which increases the per capita consumption.

This above-mentioned process in water can only be possible if there is no turbulence in the water. There are a few factors that affect the settling velocity of the water.

1. Horizontal velocity of particle which helps the particle not to settle at the bottom of the tank.
2. Shape and size of the particles
3. Viscosity of the water

Stokes law equation 1.1 and equation 1.2 for different sizes of particle to calculate the settling velocity is given below.

a) Particle diameter up to 0.1 mm

$$v_s = 418(G-1)d^2\left\{\frac{3T+70}{100}\right\} \qquad ...(1.1)$$

b) Particle diameter from 0.1 mm to 1.0 mm

$$v_s = 418(G-1)d^2\left[\frac{3T+70}{100}\right] \qquad ...(1.2)$$

Where,

v_s = Settling velocity

G = Specific density of particle

d = Diameter of the particles in mm T = temperature of water in °C

1.3.2 Variation of water demands

The consumption of water in a town is not constant for 24 hours a day it varies non-uniformly in 24 hours during day and night time. The water demands continuously rise over time. Seasonal variation also impacts the water consumption as more water is required in summer as compared to winter and rainy season. Seasonal industries also impact water demand such as crop processing industries. Daily variation occurs due to day-to-day variations in household activity. On Sundays, festivals, and holiday days the consumption of water is more than any other day.

There is also variation in hour-to-hour demands known as hourly variations. This variation is due to different water demands in the morning and evening hour as compared to the afternoon. The water consumption in the early hour of the day from 0 to 6 AM hour the water demand is very low, it increases suddenly from 6 AM to 11 AM as major domestic activity take place between these hours. After 1 PM there is reducing in demand of water as no domestic activity take place in the afternoon. Again, the water demand increases in the evening hour from 6 PM to 10 PM and finally fall to the lowest demand in the night hours as shown in figure 1.9.

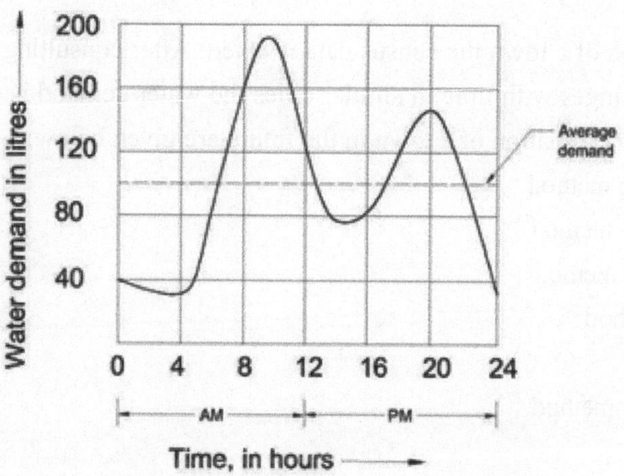

Figure 1.9: Variation in water demand

These hourly variations should be assessed properly before designing the water supply system and selecting the water sources. Suitable water demand should also be taken for firefighting demand. The maximum demand for monthly, hourly, and daily consumption is expressed in their means. The maximum hourly water demand of a town is calculated as 150% of the average hourly consumption whereas the maximum daily consumption is calculated as 180% of the average daily consumption. Therefore the maximum hourly consumption of water from a maximum daily consumption day is known as peak demand. The Government of India manual has given the peak factors value based on the population of the town as shown in Table 1.2. It can be seen from Table 1.2 that as the population increases the peak factor value decreases. It is due to presence of different cultural and habitats person in a large population which decreases the variations in demands.

Table 1.2: Peak factors based on population

S. No.	Population	Peak factor value
1	Less than 50 thousands	3.0
2	50 thousands to 2 lakhs	2.5
3	More than 2 lakhs	2.0

1.3.3 Forecasting of population

The population of a town is not constant it increases over time due to favorable conditions. Population increase will be different for different cities as it depends on the expansion of the city, electricity system, people's occupation, security of the area, etc. Transportation plays a major role in the increase in the population. In some places population also decreases due to the migration of people for better jobs, infrastructure, and safety. The Number of deaths and birth rate also affect the population of a town. Therefore the water supply system majorly depends on the right estimate of the increased population with time to get successful.

To find the exact population of a town the census data is taken. After consulting with local authorities and studying the population changes with time in similar cities the water demand is determined. Few methods to determine the population estimation of a town in the future are given below:

1. Arithmetical increase method
2. Geometrical increase method
3. Incremental increase method
4. Growth analysis method
5. Graphic method
6. Comparative graphic method
7. Zonal method

The above methods are described in the following sections.

1.3.3.1 Arithmetical Increase Method

This method is used based on certain assumptions such as the rate of increase in population is constant rate i.e. the rate at which the population changes with time remains constant. In this method, the average population of the last 3 to 5 decades is taken and an increase in population per decade is calculated. This method is used for large old city in which maximum development has taken place. The value given by this method is lower than other methods. Equation (1.3) represents the mathematical formula for the calculation arithmetical increase method.

$$P_i = \{P_a + i\bar{y}\} \qquad (1.3)$$

Where,

Pi is the forecasted population after i decade from the present population Pa is the present population

i is the number of decades for which the design population calculated

$\bar{y}$ is per decade average increase in population

Example 1.1 The population of an X town for the last 4 decades is given below. Using the arithmetical increase method find the increase in population for 2031 and 2041.

Table 1.3: Population data

Year	**Population**
1991	27,000
2001	32,000
2011	39,000
2021	48,000

Answer: The given data in table 1.3 has been extended in table 1.4 for calculate the average increase in population per decade which can be seen in column no. 4.

Table 1.4: Solution Arithmetic method

Year	**Population**	**Increase in population per decade**	**Average increase per decade**
1991	27,000	0	
2001	32,500	5500	$\frac{5500+6500+8000}{3} = 6667$
2011	39,000	6500	
2021	47,000	8000	

Forecasting population for the year 2031 and 2041 can be calculated using equation (1.3) 2031 year

$= P_{2031} = \{P_{2021} + 1 * 6667\}$

$= 47{,}000 + 6667 = 53667$ person 2041 year $= P_{2041} = \{P_{2021} + 2 * 6667\}$

$= 47000 + 13334 = 60334$ person

1.3.3.2 Geometrical Increase Method

In the geometrical increase method, the population percentage increases per decade remain constant but the increase gets compounded over the previous year every decade. The basic difference between the arithmetical increase method and the geometrical increase method is that in the first method simple arithmetic mean is taken while in the second method compounding is done for every decade. This method gives generally higher values than the arithmetical increase method. This method is used for the city which is developing at a rapid pace. Equation (1.4) represents the mathematical formula for the calculation geometrical increase method.

$$P_i = P_a\left[1+\frac{Y_b}{100}\right]^i$$

Where, Pi is the forecasted population after i decade from the present population Pa is the present population

i is the number of decades for which the design population calculated

Y_b is per decade average percentage increase in population

Example 1.2 the population of an X town for the last 4 decades is given below. Using the geometrical increase method find the increase in population for 2031 and 2041.

Table 1.3: Population data

Year	Population
1991	27,000
2001	32,000
2011	39,000
2021	48,000

Answer: The given data in table 1.3 has been extended in table 1.5 for calculate the average percentage increase in population per decade which can be seen in column no. 5.

Table 1.5: Solution Geometric method

Year	Population	Increase in population per decade	Percentage increase in population per decade	Average increase in percentage
1991	27,000	---	---	
2001	32,500	5500	$\frac{5500 \times 100}{27000} = 20.4$	$\frac{20.4 + 20 + 20.5}{3}$
2011	39,000	6500	$\frac{6500 \times 100}{32500} = 20$	= 20.3
2021	47,000	8000	$\frac{8000 \times 100}{39000} = 20.5$	

Forecasting population for the years 2031 and 2041 can be calculated using equation (1.4)

$$2031 \text{ year} = P_{2031} = P_{2021}\left[1+\frac{20.3}{100}\right]^1$$

$$= 47000\times1.203 = 56541 \text{ person}$$

$$2041 \text{ year} = P_{2041} = P_{2021}\left[1+\frac{20.3}{100}\right]^2$$

$$= 47000\times(1.203)^2 = 47000\times1.4472 = 68019 \text{ Person}$$

1.3.3.3 Incremental Increase Method

In this method the population increase rate for per decade not remain constant as the case in arithmetical increase method and geometrical increase method. It depends on the incremental increase on the average increase in population per decade. It can be positive or negative. This method gives the value in between the geometrical increase method and the arithmetical increase method. In this method first, the average increase in population per decade is calculated in the same way as in method 1. Then the incremental increase in the average increase is calculated and it's added to it. This method can be used for any type of town old or new. Equation (1.5) represents the mathematical formula for the calculation geometrical increase method.

$$P_i = P_a + (N_a + N_b)i \qquad (1.5)$$

Where,

Pi is the forecasted population after i decade from the present population Pa is the present population

i is the number of decades for which the design population calculated

N_b is incremental increase over average increase in population per decade

Example 1.3 The population of an X town for the last 4 decades is given below. Using the geometrical increase method find the increase in population for 2031 and 2041.

Table 1.3 Population data

Year	Population
1991	27,000
2001	32,000
2011	39,000
2021	48,000

Answer: The given data in Table 1.3 has been extended in Table 1.6 for calculate the average increase in population per decade which can be seen in column no. 3 and incremental increase over average increase can be seen in column no. 4.

Table 1.6: Solution Incremental Increase method

Year	Population	Increase in population per decade	Percentage increase in population per decade
1991	27,000	---	---
2001	32,500	5500	---
2011	39,000	6500	6500 – 5500 = 1000
2021	47,000	8000	8000 – 6500 = 1500
	Total	20000	2500
	Average	20000/3 = 6667	2500/2 = 1250

Forecasting population for the year 2031 and 2041 can be calculated using equation (1.5) 2031 year = P_{2031} = $\{P_{2021} + (6667 + 1250) \times 1\}$

= 47,000 + 7917 = 54917 person

2041 year = $P_{2041} = \{P_{2021} + (6667 + 1250) \times 2\}$

= 47000 + 15834 = 62834 person

1.3.3.4 Growth Analysis Method

In this method the natural factors due to which population increase or decrease are taken into consideration. These factors are birth rate of a town and death rate of a town. The difference between death rate and birth rate gives the natural growth rate of the town. Positive increase in the population in a town occur when there birth rate is more than the death rate while negative growth rate occur when vice-versa occurs. Migrations of population on a large scale also affect the natural growth of a town. It can be positive when the population from outside settles in a town and can be negative if the people move out of the town. Equation (1.6) can be adopted for calculating the natural growth of a population of a town.

$$P_i = [(P_a \times Y_a) - (P_a \times Y_b)]i \qquad (1.6)$$

Where,

Pi is the forecasted population after i decade from the present population Pa is the present population

i is the number of decades for which the design population calculated

Y_a is per decade birth rate

Y_b is per decade death rate

1.3.3.5 Graphical Method

In graphical method the graph is plotted against the population and time from the available data. From the plotted graph the line is extended to the desired design period and the approximate population against that design period can be calculated. In this method, the extension of curve is depend on the person capability and if it's not done carefully it can give the wrong estimation of the population. Figure 1.10 shows graphs plotted using data from table 1.3. From this graph we can calculate the population for 2031 year which is around 54000 and for 2041 year is 62000.

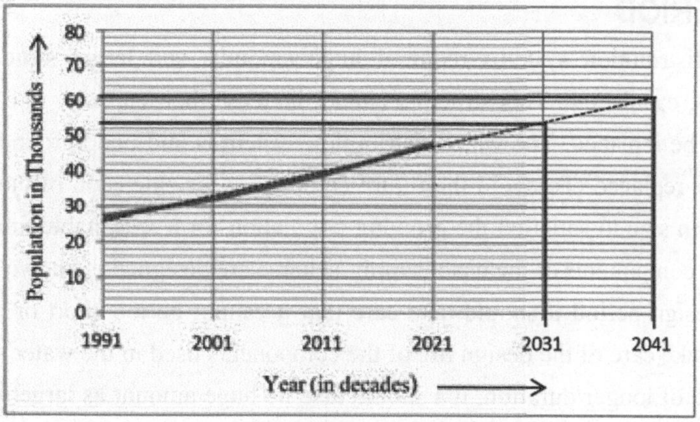

Figure 1.10: Graphical Method

1.3.3.6 Comparative Graphical Method

In comparative graphical method the city is selected which have similar conditions and characteristics to the proposed city for which future population has to be estimated. In this method, the population determined is correct as the statistics data of the developed city is similar to the proposed city. For this method, it becomes difficult to find the city having similar equality data and characteristics data.

1.3.3.7 Comparative Graphical Method

Nowadays larger and bigger cities are generally developed by the planning department of a state. While developing city the maximum population is estimated per hectare. The area of the town is designated according to the uses such as commercial and residential uses. The expansion of a town is governed by certain by-laws of local development authority. Only development can occur which is planned in the master plan of the town. In a master plan the future population is estimated and accordingly the water supply scheme is designed. In this method, the population density of an area is fixed. With the help of master plan its gives the location where the residential plots and industrial area will get established. Table 1.7 gives the population density per hectare for different categories in a master plan.

Table 1.7: Population density per hectare according to area

S. No.	Area types	Population density per hectare
1	Residential area: a. Single-family or multiple-family houses	40 – 250
	b. Multi-story Apartments	More than 250
2	Commercial/Business areas	40 - 75
3	Industrial hubs	10 - 40

1.3.4 DESIGN PERIOD

While laying water distribution systems required huge amounts and larger structures such as dams, reservoirs, waterworks, canals, etc. This structure cannot increase their capacity in conveniently and easy ways and they cannot be replaced. The water distribution system is laid underground by digging the road and it cannot be easily replaced. To avoid the future complexity for extension of these water distribution system for laid larger in size to satisfied the growing population for a reasonable time period. This future year for which various components of the water supply scheme are designed is known as the design period. While deciding the design period it should take care that it cannot be too short or too long. The design period should always take care of the design life of the components used in the water supply scheme. If we choose a design period of longer duration, it's should also be huge amount as larger water treatment units to be made and bigger diameter pipes to be installed which will unnecessary increase the burden on the present population. Water distribution system for generally circumstance should be taken for 30 year (Water Supply and Drainage handbook (SP 35: 1987) of BIS) of design period. This design period starts after the completion of the project. Provision for the expansion of the project in the future the necessary arrangement of land should be done before starting the project. According to Ministry of Housing and Urban Affairs, Government of India, manual on water supply and treatment systems (2023) the designed period for various components are shown in table no 1.8.

1.3.5 Estimating of quantity of water supply required for a city or town

It is difficult to precisely estimate the quality of water supply required for a city or town as it depends on many factors that affect water consumption. There are certain empirical formulas and thumb rules which give quite accurate results. The uses of this formula depend on the intelligence of the person who is using it to calculate the water supply demand. The various water demands that affect a city or town's requirements are

1. Domestic purpose
2. Commercial and industrial purpose
3. Public use
4. Firefighting demand
5. Water losses in wastage and thefts

Table 1.8: Design periods for various components of the water distribution scheme

S. No.	Various item list	Design periods (year)
1	Water storage by reservoir/dams/ weirs	50
2	Intakes and jacks well a. Pump house b. electric work	50 15

3	Waterworks units	15
4	Distribution pipes in the treatment of water in the water treatment plant	15
5	The distribution system contains raw and treated water	30
6	Water treatment plants clear reservoir	15
7	Tube wells and bore wells (groundwater source)	15

1.3.5.1 DOMESTIC PURPOSE

This demand includes the water used for residential purposes such as bathing, cooking, washing, drinking, sprinkling of water in lawns, sanitary systems, gardening, etc. The variation in water demand for particular persons depends on their living standards. According to Indian standard code 1172-1993 (reaffirmed 2007) mentioned the water demand for per person per day is 135 lpcd. Its breakdown is shown below and units are lpcd:

a) Drinking purpose	5
b) Bathing Purpose	55
c) Cloth washing	20
d) Utensil washing	10
e) Food preparation	5
f) Housing cleaning and floor washing	10
g) Sanitary flushing system	30
Total	135

Domestic water consumption compromises of 50% to 60% of the total demand of a city or town. In developed country such as USA or European Union the water demand is more than 340 lpcd it is because they used more water as per there living standards such as tub bathing, dish washers, car washing etc.

1.3.5.2 Commercial and industrial demand

In industrial water demand it represents all the demand necessary for the existing industries and the industries likely to be setup in the design period. This demand may vary on types and nature of industries present in the city. The water demand for ordinary industries is taken as 50 lpcd, which is only for the small industries present in the town and it do not involve the demand for large industries. Table 1.9 shows the water demand for various industries. Some large industries make their own facilities to meet the water demand and they do not depend on public water demand.

Commercial water demand also depends on the nature and type of commercial hub present in the city. In general, around 20 lpcd is sufficient to meet the requirement of commercial area but in a city where highly commercial activities take place, this demand can reach up to 50 lpcd.

Table 1.9: Various industries' water demand

S. No.	Type of industry	Water demand based on per unit production in liters
1	Sugar cane industry	15000 - 25000 per tonne
2	Oil refinery industry	2000 - 3000 per tonne
3	Paper industry	200000 - 400000 per tonne
4	Leather industry	40000 – 60000 per tonne
5	Textile Industry	80000 – 140000 per tonne

1.3.5.3 Public Use

This water demand includes the water requirement for public uses such as fountains in parks, watering of public gardens, washing and water sprinkling on road, etc. This water demand is not considered essential in most of the cities in India and there is generally taken as less than 5% of the total demand. In generally an amount of 10 lpcd is added in the water demand for a city or town as public uses.

1.3.5.4 Firefighting demand

Fire generally breaks out in larger and thickly populated towns due to electric short circuits, leakage from gas cylinder, and other reasons. Larger cities have their firefighting team which requires a large amount of water to dispose of the fire. In modern cities, there should be provision for firefighting in the water supply system. This amount should be easily available for fire extinguishers and always stored in the fire station in their reservoir. The water requirement is for a short duration of 4 to 5 hours but the amount of water required is high with good pressure in the fire hydrant.

There are different empirical formulas to calculate the water demand and rate of flow of water to get fire extinguish. These formulas depend on the number of populations in a city. Few are described below with equation no. (1.7), (1.8), (1.9), and (1.10), where Q = water required in liters per minute, P = Population per thousand for all equations mentioned below

(i) Kuichling formula:

$$Q = 3182\sqrt{P} \tag{1.7}$$

(ii) John Ripley Freeman formula:

$$Q = 1136\left\{\frac{P}{5} + 10\right\} \tag{1.8}$$

(iii) Boston formula:

$$Q = 5663\sqrt{P} \tag{1.9}$$

(iv) National Board of Fire under-writers formula:

$$Q = 4637\sqrt{P}[1 - 0.01\sqrt{P}] \tag{1.10}$$

These empirical formulas will remain same for every area and location because in these formulas the type of location, public density, industrial areas are not considered. Commercial and industrial areas are very prone to catch fire. While using the above formulas and converted into lpcd its value for Indian condition comes less than 1 lpcd. Fire hydrants are provided on the main distribution line at the junction and intersection of the city or some important points. These hydrants should be capable of handling a pressure of 1.5 kg/cm^2 and can supply non-interfering water for 4 to 5 hours.

1.3.5.5 Water losses in wastage and thefts

In larger cities having higher water distribution pressures the losses due to leakage increase and thefts from the main distribution pipe line. Due to this a large amount of water is wasted and its counts for about 15% to 40% of the total water supply of a city. This waste can be reduced by proper joints but not be completely controlled.

1.4 QUALITY OF WATER

The pure form of water does not exist on Earth. Water formed by an experimental process in the laboratory by lighting the hydrogen molecules with oxygen molecules in a test tube is not guaranteed to be the purest form as it may contain glass particles. As in the case of precipitation at the times of making rainfall the water is in pure form but when its fall down on earth it mixes with different gases and impurities. After falling on the earth surface it gets mixed with soil impurities of biological and non-biological. While running on the surface of earth it gets in contact with garbage, pesticides, and animal waste. Different types of impurities get dissolved in water when its pass through different aquifers while traveling underground The water gets dissolved with heavy metals and toxic chemicals such as lead, arsenic, chromium, etc. which are very dangerous for human beings. These different types of impurities in the water can cause waterborne diseases such as cholera, typhoid, and hepatitis.

For the safety of human beings and proper utilization of water in the industries, the engineering and planner while developing a water supply scheme ensure the quality, safety, and proper treatment of raw water to have desired and safe value to ensure the safety of human beings. Water supply is done for domestic purposes such as drinking, cooking, and bathing then the analysis becomes more important before distributing the water.

1.4.1 NEED FOR ANALYSIS OF WATER

The need for analysis of water is to meet the safety standard prescribed by the stationary bodies and adhere to norms and procedures to provide contamination-free water. It's a broad process in which several parameters are checked and analyzed for the quality of the water.

Water which is used for domestic and industrial purpose must be analysis regularly to protect the source of the water and free from environmental hazardous and to protect the human beings from water borne disease. With the help of analysis of water we get the information about the type of contamination and proper treatment process developed to remove the contamination. It is vital to analyze the water quality before supply. Water analysis helps in deciding the uses of water.

1.4.2 CHARACTERISTICS OF WATER

The treated water before supplying to a city is checked for physical, chemical and biological characteristics. Each of these characteristics is explained in the below section.

1.4.2.1 Physical Characteristics

In orders to determine the physical characteristics of the water different physical properties are analyses. These different properties are temperature, turbidity, taste, color, etc.

i. **Temperature:** Temperature of water is analyzed at the sources using probes which consist of thermometer. Temperatures generally do not affect the water quality as we cannot control the temperature at the source or during supply. The desired temperature for a water supply is below 10°C while the temperature above 30°C is objectionable. Higher temperature helps in dissolving the impurities which is not good for portable water.

ii. **Taste and odor:** Dissolved inorganic minerals, organic matter and dissolved gases impart taste and odour to the water. Different gas which is dissolved in water such as hydrogen sulfide, methane, carbon dioxide, etc. present with organic matter imparts different types of taste to the water. Taste and odour of the water is classified to salty or bitter, sweet, pungent smell and ordinary smell by testing and smelling of water. The odor and taste of water depend on the individual. Osmoscope device is used for measuring odour and it's measured in threshold number. A threshold number less than 3 is acceptable for water supply.

iii. **Color:** Dissolved inorganic minerals and salts, organic matter such as decaying leaves and vegetation imparts natural color to the water. The green color of the water is generally imparted due to the excessive growth of microorganisms such as microalgae. Color in the water is not objectionable due to health reason but it can spoil the color of the water clothes if we washed using color water. People do not like to drink colored water due to aesthetics and physiological reasons. Color in the water is measured by comparing it with the platinum-cobalt scale. Platinum- cobalt scale is formed by mixing one milligram of platinum-cobalt in one liter of distilled water. This mixture formed is measured as one part per million (ppm) or one mg/liter. Different intensities of color samples are made by dissolving 2mg, 3mg, 4 mg, and so on to form 2 ppm, 3 ppm, 4 ppm, and so on. For domestic water supply scheme the maximum color intensity should not be more than 20.

iv. **Turbidity:** Turbidity in the water is due to the presence of dissolved organic matter, and suspended and colloidal impurities such as sand, silt, or clay. The value of turbidity depends on the concentration of impurities present in the water. Turbid water cannot use for drinking purpose due to psychological reason but it do not have any health related issues.

As people do not want to drink turbid water, the turbidity of water should be removed to the permissible limit prescribed by the government. The turbidity of water is measured using a turbidity rod or by-passing light rays through the water and the resistance created by water is measured. Their unit is ppm. The standard for measuring and comparing turbidity water is made by dissolving finely powdered silica of one milligram in one liter of distilled water to formed one ppm unit. The permissible unit of turbidity for drinking water should be less than 10 ppm. A turbidity rod is used to measure turbidity in the field while turbid meters are used to measure turbidity in the laboratory.

1.4.2.2 Chemical Characteristics

To determine the chemical characteristics of the water different chemical properties are analyzed. These different properties are total solids, chlorides, fluoride, pH, nitrogen and its compounds, hardness, dissolved oxygen, etc.

i. **Total Solids:** Suspended and dissolved solids together form total solids in water. To determine total solids in water a known quantity of water sample is taken in bowl and it is placed in a heating oven at a temperature of 105°C to evaporate the water. The weight of the dried bowl is taken. Suspended solids can be measured by filtering the known quantity of water and measuring the residue weight on filter paper. Dissolved solids are measured by subtracting the suspended solids from total solids. The measuring unit is ppm. The permissible limit of total solids in drinking water as per IS code is 500 ppm and the maximum limit is 2000 ppm.

ii. **pH:** pH value represents the hydrogen ion concentration in water. With the help of pH, we can know whether the water is acidic or alkaline. pH of water can be measured by the logarithm of the reciprocal of hydrogen ions as shown in equation no. 1.11. This means higher the value of hydrogen ions in water the lesser the value of pH which represents the acidic nature of water and vice-versa represents the alkaline nature of water.

$$pH = log\left(\frac{1}{H^+}\right) \qquad ...(1.11)$$

In distilled water the number of positive charge hydrogen ions and negative charge hydroxyl ions are equal in number and it makes the water neutral. pH of water at neutral condition is 7, if the pH value is more than 7 it is alkaline with maximum value at pH 14. If the pH value is less than 7 it is acidic with a maximum value of 0 values. It means a pH scale varies from 0 to 14. To calculate the pH of water, the sample is compared to the pre- mix standard solution of known pH by adding an indicator to the sample. This process is known as the calorimetric method. Another method by which the pH of a water sample is calculated is known as a potentiometer. In this method, the electric potential is measured due to the presence of hydrogen ions and their concentration. pH value display in the digital display device.

iii. **Chlorides:** Chloride is the most commonly found element in groundwater and it is often formed in compound forms with sodium, potassium, or calcium. In groundwater, chloride is present due to geological formation containing salts, contribution from wastewater, or the intrusion of salty water into the ground. Chloride in the water sample is calculated by the Mohr method. In this method the sample is titrated using silver nitrate, an indicator i.e. potassium chromate is used to know the endpoints. In this method, during titration, the sample color changes to a reddish-brown precipitate, which means all the chloride consumed and the burette reading gives the chloride content. The maximum permissible value of chloride in water as per IS code is 200 ppm.

iv. **Hardness:** The hardness in the water prevents the formation of the foam. The main reason of hardness in water is present of salts of calcium and magnesium with carbonate, bi- carbonate, sulfate and chloride. This salt makes a layer on the surface of soap which prevents to form foam. Hard water do not used in domestic and industrial purpose as it leads to increase in consumption of soap, corrosion and scaling of boiler and produces salty taste in food. Hardness is expressed in ppm.

Hardness can be classified into two parts:

a. **Carbonate hardness:** This type of hardness is due to the presence of salts of carbonate and bi-carbonate with calcium and magnesium. It is also known as temporary hardness, because this hardness can be removed by boiling. When we boil the water it forms the precipitation of calcium carbonate and magnesium carbonate which settle at the bottom of the pan. The color of precipitation is white in color.

b. **Non-carbonate hardness:** this type of hardness is due to the presence of salts of sulfate and chloride with calcium and magnesium in water. It is also known as permanent hardness. As this hardness cannot remove by boiling they require some special process to remove the hardness and to make water soft. Different chemical processes are used to remove permanent hardness. Some of them are the lime and soda ash process, zeolite process etc.

Hardness in water in the laboratory can be calculated by using versenate method. In this process, ethylene di-amine tetra-citric acid is used for titration of water sample. Indicator used for titration is erio-chrome black T- indicator. In this water is titrating till the water sample color changes from red to blue. Burette reading gives the hardness of water.

v. **Fluoride:** Fluoride minerals naturally occurred in the ground water due to presence of fluoride minerals ore which release fluoride in water as water passes through this ores. Some quantity of fluoride is required by our body as it prevents decaying of tooth and makes them stronger. As per IS the desired limit of fluoride is 1 mg/l and the maximum permissible limit is 1.5 mg/l.

Fluoride in water can be measured by electrochemical probe and chemical method in laboratory. In chemical method zirconium alizarin regent is used in which red color is changed into orange-yellow color and matched with the fluoride standard already made of different strength. In this method the maximum concentration in which fluoride is measured is 1 mg/l and the least value is 0.05 mg/l. In electrochemical method the fluoride ions selective electrode is used. The fluoride value it can detect in the range from 0.2 mg/l to 2 g/l.

vi. **Nitrogen and its compounds:** In water, if nitrogen is present it will indicate the presence of organic water. The water run-off from the agricultural field is also the main factor due to which nitrogen compounds found in water. Different forms in which nitrogen found in water are ammonia nitrogen, nitrates, nitrites and organic nitrogen.

In water if there is ammonia nitrogen is presents it indicates the decaying of organic matter and during decaying the free ammonia is released. Free ammonia in water indicates the recent pollution in water. Ammonia nitrogen permissible value as per IS code is less than 0.15 mg/l. It can be measured in laboratory by distillation process. In this process the water is boiled and the release ammonia is measured.

Organic nitrogen in water indicates the amount of nitrogen in the form of un-decaying organic matter which releases ammonia when digested. Organic nitrogen vale as per IS code should not be more than 0.3 mg/l in water. It can be calculated by digestion of un- decayed organic matter and measuring the amount of ammonia released. In the digestion process, potassium permanganate is added to the water which is already boiled and after adding potassium permanganate it is again boiled and the release of ammonia is measured.

The ammonia nitrogen and organic nitrogen together in water is known as Kjedahl nitrogen. If nitrites are present in water it indicates the partial decomposition of organic water. It is highly poisonous to the human body. Its recommended value as per IS code is nil. If nitrates are present in water it indicates the complete decomposition of organic matter. It is not harmful for human beings but if nitrates are present in large quantities in water it affects the infants causing blue baby diseases. The maximum amount of nitrates in water as per IS code is 45 mg/l. Both nitrites and nitrates in water are measured by using color matching method. Nitrogen in any form present in water indicates it has been contaminated with domestic wastewater or any organic waste. A different form of nitrogen also helps in knowing the time the water gets contaminated.

vii. **Dissolved oxygen:** Oxygen gas gets dissolved in the water through the atmosphere. Due to the presence of oxygen in the water, it remains fresh. The amount of oxygen above saturation level in water is harmful for industrial and domestic purposes as it can cause rusting of the pipeline. If there is a low amount of oxygen in water it can indicate that the water contains organic matter as oxygen is consumed by bacteria for the decomposition of organic matter. The measurement of dissolved oxygen is done using modified wrinkle methods. Cold water has more amount of saturated oxygen as compared to warm water. The maximum value of dissolved oxygen in water can be attained at 0°C i.e. 14.6 mg/l and as the temperature increases this value decreases at 20°C and 30°C the saturation dissolved oxygen is 9.1 mg/l and 7.0 mg/l respectively.

1.4.2.3 Biological Characteristics

Surface water contains different types of bacteria. These bacteria come in contact with water from sewage and household waste. Bacteria in water are of different shapes and sizes having a single cell with no chlorophyll material that depends on others for food. The size of bacteria varies from 0.2 μm to 5 μm. Bacteria size is so small they cannot be seen by the naked eye which a microscope has to be used to see. Their growth is done by binary fusion and very fast.

Some bacteria are not harmful to human beings and animals. These bacteria are known as non- pathogenic bacteria. Bacteria which are harmful to human beings and animals and cause harmful waterborne diseases are known as pathogenic bacteria. During the treatment of water for water supply, the pathogenic bacteria are only removed.

Most of bacteria present in water require oxygen for their growth and decomposed organic matter for their food. They consume oxygen from dissolved oxygen in water. These types of bacteria which consume oxygen are known as aerobic bacteria. While some bacteria survived without oxygen in water. They are known as anaerobic bacteria. There is one another type of bacteria present in water which can survive in both oxygen and no oxygen conditions. They are known as facultative bacteria.

1.4.3 Bacteriological test

Bacteriological tests are done to find the pathogenic and non-pathogenic bacteria in water. The tests on pathogenic bacteria are very lengthy and complicated. So, we regularly do not perform this type of test on the water to check their quality. Tests are generally done to check the pathogenic bacteria which can be done easily. The primary nonpathogenic bacteria that are detected is coliform. Coliform bacteria if present in water it indicates the water is contaminated with sewage waste which confirms the presence of pathogen bacteria in water. Coliform bacteria are present in the colon of human beings and are found in feces of human. Coliform bacteria consist of total coliform, fecal coliform.

1.4.4 E-Coli

Escherichia coli are also known as E-coli are a type of fecal coliform whose presence indicates feces of human. E-coli is only coliform which can only live in the intestine of human beings and animals. Test of E-coli confirms that water was recently contaminated with sewage waste. The most important and simple method by which E-coli are detected in water is passing the water through a sterile membrane having pores size of 5 μm to 10 μm. Then this filter paper is placed in M-Endo's broth or LES Endo agar which is suitable nutrients for E-coli growth and incubated at 37°C. E-coli bacteria will grow and visible colonies (pink to dark red color) will be produced and counted. Each counted colony represents one bacterium in the original sample. These processes are known as culturing bacteria through culture medium.

1.4.5 B-coli Index

B-coli are from the bacillus colon group. B-coli is also present in the intestines of human beings and animals. Their number varies from a few hundred to very low based on the contamination of water from pollution. B-coli in water can be determined by following a few steps:

- **Step 1:** This step is known as a preliminary test which indicates that B-coli bacteria is present in water or not. In this test, lactose broth is incubated with the water sample and kept at 37°C for 24 hr. in an incubation chamber. After completion of time, the gas is seen in the test tube. If the amount of gas is present in the test tube it indicates that B-coli bacteria are present in the sample.
- **Step 2:** In this step the positive tube broth is transferred into another broth which is lactose bile green in color. If after 48 hours gas is visible in this broth the final step will be concluded. This step confirms the presence of B-coli.

AICTE'S LIST OF PRESCRIBED TEXTBOOKS

As Per Model Curriculum & Outcome Based Education

aligned with

NATIONAL EDUCATION POLICY 2020

UNDERGRADUATE COURSE BOOKS

S.No.	ISBN	Book Name	Author
1	9789355382160	Advanced Electrical Machines: Theory and Practicals	Bharat Singh Rajpurohit
2	9789355382139	Analog Electronic Circuits: Theory and Practical	Venu Sonti, Sachin Jain
3	9789355383808	Analog Electronic Devices: Theory and Practicals	N. B Balamurugan
4	9789391505158	Basic Electrical Engineering (with Lab Manual)	S.K. Sahdev
5	9789355388087	Basic of Electronics	Brijesh Iyer
6	9789355387127	Basics of Electrical Machines: Theory and Practicals	D. K. Palwalia, U. K. Kalla, R. K. Kumawat
7	9789355389381	Basics of Mechanics	Shubhankar Bhowmick, N. Venkata Swamy Naidu
8	9789355386250	Basics of Thermodynamics	Parmod Kumar, Atul Dhar
9	9789355386984	Biology for Engineers	Annamma Odaneth
10	9789391505141	Chemistry-I	Manisha Agarwal
11	9789355384843	Civil Engineering Societal and Global Impact	Shakuntala Acharya
12	9789355382184	Computer Aided Civil Engineering Drawing	D. Chandra Mouli, B. Swathi
13	9789355382580	Computer Aided Design & Analysis	Hari Kumar Voruganti
14	9789355387592	Computer Architecture	D. Vaithiyanathan
15	9789355385093	Computer Networks	Hari Prabhat Gupta
16	9789355385307	Construction Engineering & Management	Sparsh Johari
17	9789355388728	Control Systems	S.N. Deepa
18	9789355385420	Data Structure and Algorithms	Ranbir Singh Sanasam
19	9789355386700	Design and Analysis of Algorithms	Hari P. Gupta, Rahul Mishra
20	9789355388872	Digital Electronics and System	Abhishek Bhatt
21	9789355386571	Digital Signal Processing	Sanjeev Sharma
22	9789355383396	Disaster management	Pradeep K. Goyal, Anil K. Gupta
23	9789355385222	Discrete Mathematical Structures	Narendra S. Chaudhari, Sharmila S. P.
24	9789355387868	Effective Technical Communication	Pritee Sharma, Sanchita Verma
25	9789355383389	Electrical Circuit Analysis and Network Theory	Shouri Chatterjee
26	9789355388957	Electromagnetic Waves	Uttam M. Pal, Srijith K.
27	9789355384652	Electronic Communication	Vimal Bhatia
28	9789355388711	Embedded Systems	Santanu Chattopadhyay
29	9789355385147	Energy Science and Engineering	M. Rizwan, Majid Jamil
30	9789355387929	Engineering Economics, Estimation & Costing	Yogesh C. Joshi
31	9789355384669	Engineering Geology	R. N. Khare, Ketan Chourasia
32	9789391505066	Engineering Graphics & Design	Pradeep Jain
33	9789391505097	English (with Lab Manual)	Kulbhushan Kumar
34	9789355385963	Environmental Engineering	Chandra Sekhar Matli
35	9789355388117	Fluid Mechanics	Shreenivas N. Londhe, Pradnya R. Dixit
36	9789355388377	Fluid Mechanics & Fluid Machines	R.P. Saini
37	9789355387103	Geotechnical Engineering	Paramita Bhattacharya

UNDERGRADUATE COURSE BOOKS

S.No.	ISBN	Book Name	Author
38	9789355385130	Hydraulic Engineering	Sayantan Ganguly
39	9789355385550	Hydrology & Water Resources Engineering	Mitthan Lal Kansal, P.K. Agarwal
40	9789355389688	Information Technology Workshop in MATLAB	Hari Prabhat Gupta
41	9789355383235	Instrumentation for Civil Engineering Applications	Ashim Kanti Dey, Manita Das
42	9789355387042	Introduction to Civil Engineering	Manabendra Saharia, Nagendra R. Velaga
43	9789355384805	Introduction to Database Systems	Vikram Singh
44	9789355387509	Machine Element & System Design	Sabah Khan
45	9789355385383	Machine Learning	Himanshu Mittal
46	9789355388414	Manufacturing Automation	Chitragupt Swaroop Chitransh
47	9789355387233	Manufacturing Processes	Dheerendra Kumar Dwivedi
48	9789355389886	Materials Engineering	Dheerendra Kumar Dwivedi
49	9789391505172	Mathematics - I Calculus and Linear Algebra [For Non-Computer Science Engineering Branches]	Reena Garg
50	9789391505271	Mathematics - I Calculus and Linear Algebra [For Computer Science Engineering Branches]	Reena Garg
51	9789355384607	Measurements & Metrology	V.P. Chandramohan
52	9789355383730	Mechanics of Materials	Arvind Vyavahare
53	9789355383358	Mechatronics, Robotics & Control	J. Srinivas
54	9789355385116	Microprocessor and Microcontroller	Saurabh Chaudhury, Risha Mal
55	9789355386083	Microprocessors	Yogendra Kumar Gupta
56	9789355389169	Mobile Communication and Networks	Vimal Bhatia
57	9789355385475	Operating Systems	Sukomal Pal
58	9789355385604	Operating Systems	Sanjaya Kumar Panda
59	9789391505134	Physics (Oscillations, Waves and Optics) With lab manual	A.B. Bhattacharya, Atanu Nag
60	9789391505257	Physics (Quantum Mechanics for Engineers) With lab manual	A.B. Bhattacharya, Atanu Nag
61	9789391505165	Physics (Introduction to Electromagnetic Theory) (with Lab Manual)	A.B. Bhattacharya, Atanu Nag
62	9789391505059	Physics (Introduction to Mechanics) (with Lab Manual)	A.B. Bhattacharya, Atanu Nag
63	9789355385956	Power Electronics: Theory and Practicals	Lalit Chandra Saikia
64	9789355384942	Power Systems-I	Suresh Mikkili
65	9789355386236	Power Systems-II	Arun Rahul S, Manas K. Jena
66	9789355383754	Product Innovation & Entrepreneurship	Vigneswaran C
67	9789355384584	Production & Operation Management	Navin Kumar Dev
68	9789391505219	Programming for Problem Solving (with Lab Manual)	R.S. Salaria
69	9789355385451	Signals and Systems	Sanjay L. Nalbalwar
70	9789355386021	Strength of Materials	Uday Shanker Dixit, Nelson Muthu, S. M. Kamal
71	9789355383792	Structural Engineering	T.D. Gunneswara Rao, D. Ravi Prasad
72	9789355387004	Surveying and Geomatics	P. K. Garg
73	9789355384317	Testing & Evaluation of Civil Engineering Materials	Sandeep Chaudhary, Kashyap A Patel
74	9789355382306	Theory of Computation	Debi Prasanna Acharjya
75	9789355384928	Transportation Engineering	A.K. Raji
76	9789355385208	VLSI Design	Mahendra Sakare, Shonal Chouksey
77	9789391505332	Workshop / Manufacturing Practices (with Lab Manual)	Veeranna D.K.

DIPLOMA COURSE BOOKS

S.No.	ISBN	Book Name	Author
1	9789355382481	Aanandam An Act of Community Service	Shuchi Sharma
2	9789355385567	Advanced Manufacturing Processes	Ranjeet Kumar Sahu, Devendra Laxman Kamble
3	9789355385109	Advanced Surveying: Theory & Practice	Ramakant Agrawal, Parshottam Sarathe
4	9789355384546	Algorithms	Piyoosh P, Arnab Sarkar
5	9789391505448	Applied Chemistry (with Lab Manual)	Anju Rawlley, Devdatta Vinayakrao Saraf
6	9789391505431	Applied Physics-I (with Lab Manual)	Vinod Kumar Yadav, Mina Talati
7	9789391505578	Applied Physics-II (with Lab Manual)	Hussain Jeevakhan
8	9789355387530	Basic Mechanical Engineering	Dharmendra Singh, Chandra Shekhar Rajoria
9	9789355387394	Building Construction	Rinku Kumar, Sandeep Panchal
10	9789355383280	Building Electrification	Arnab Ghosh
11	9789355384379	Building Planning and Drawing	Aparna Dwivedi
12	9789391505493	Communication Skills in English	Anjana Tiwari
13	9789355383570	Computer Aided Machine Drawing Practice	Kanak Kalita
14	9789355388964	Computer Networking and Data Communication	Sanjaya Shankar Tripathy
15	9789355382986	Computer Networks: Theory & Practicals	Brijendra Pratap Singh, Manoj Madhava Gore
16	9789355382672	Computer Programming: Theory and Practicals	Satyendra Singh Chouhan
17	9789355387714	Computer System Organization	Sonal Yadav
18	9789355382658	Concrete Technology: Theory and Practice	Sasankasekhar Mandal, Vishwajit Anand, Sushil K. Agarwala
19	9789355383334	Construction Materials and Testing	Vanita Aggarwal
20	9789355383501	Consumer Electronics	Amit M. Joshi, Maulin M. Joshi, Urvashi Prakash Shukla
21	9789355387684	Data Structures: Theory & Practicals	NB Venkateswarlu
22	9789355388513	Design of Machine Elements	A. Kumaravel, M. Kathirselvam
23	9789355388360	Design of Steel and RCC Structure	Sparsh Johari
24	9789355383303	Digital Communication	Muralidhar Kulkarni, K. S. Shivaprakasha
25	9789355387295	Digital Electronics	Menka Yadav
26	9789355389435	Electric Circuits and Networks	Jamuna K., Nilanjan Tewari
27	9789355388452	Electric Motors and Transformers (Theory and Practicals)	Sanjay B. Bodkhe
28	9789355385901	Electric Power Transmission and Distribution	Sudhir Sharma
29	9789355389466	Electrical & Electronics Measurements and Instrumentation	Sudarsan Sahoo, Vipin Chandra Pal, Sudipta Chakraborty
30	9789355382696	Electronic Communication	M. D. Selvaraj, P. Nagaradjane
31	9789355387202	Electronic Devices and Circuits	Ankesh Jain
32	9789355386373	Electronic Equipment Maintenance	Chanchal Sharma
33	9789355384690	Embedded Systems	Deepa M, G. Santhanamari, Susithra. N
34	9789355384867	Energy Conservation and Audit	M. Rizwan, Majid Jamil
35	9789391505509	Engineering Graphics	Sharad K. Pradhan, K.K. Jain
36	9789391505608	Engineering Mechanics (with Lab Manual)	Bhankhar Bharat, Gokaldas Vandana Somkuwar

DIPLOMA COURSE BOOKS

S.No.	ISBN	Book Name	Author
37	9789391505516	Engineering Workshop Practice	A. K. Sarathe
38	9789391505653	Environmental Science	Subrat Roy
39	9789355384966	Estimating, Costing and valuation	Sandeep Panchal
40	9789355389510	Fluid Mechanics & Hydraulic Machinery	Suman Chakraborty, Sourav Mitra, Aditya Bandopadhyay
41	9789391505592	Fundamentals of Electrical and Electronics Engineering (with Lab Manual)	Susan S. Mathew, Saji T. Chacko
42	9789355387240	Fundamentals of Power Electronics	Soumitra Kumar Mandal
43	9789355389602	Geotechnical Engineering (Theory & Practicals)	Neelima Satyam
44	9789355386137	Induction, Synchronous, and Special Electrical Machines	K. Selvajyothi, S. Tamilselvi, Sarat Kumar Sahoo
45	9789355382290	Industrial Engineering & Management	A. Manimaran
46	9789355384959	Internet of Things	Sujata Pal
47	9789355388650	Introduction to DBMS: Theory & Practicals	Myneni Madhu Bala
48	9789355384294	Introduction to e-Governance	Kamal Kant Verma
49	9789355386564	Introduction to Electric Generation Systems	Lalit Chandra Saikia, Nalin Behari, Deb Choudhury
50	9789391505585	Introduction to IT Systems (with Lab Manual)	Prashant Joshi
51	9789355382900	Linear Integrated Circuit	B. T. Krishna
52	9789355388148	Manufacturing Engineering	Santosh Kumar
53	9789355383877	Material Science & Engineering	Vinod Kumar, Nisheeth k. Prasad
54	9789391505424	Mathematics-I	Deepak Singh
55	9789391505523	Mathematics-II	Garima Singh
56	9789355385994	Measurements and Metrology	A. Gnanavelbabu, M. Santhana kumar, R. Saranraj
57	9789355388131	Mechanics of Materials and their Testing	R. Velmurugan, Pragathi
58	9789355385048	Microcontroller Applications	Ritula Thakur
59	9789355385062	Microcontrollers and Applications	Santanu Chattopadhyay
60	9789355388100	Mobile and Wireless Communication	Maulin Joshi, Urvashi P. Shukla
61	9789355387790	Production & Operations Management	Mayank Kumar Agrawal
62	9789355388704	Public Health Engineering	Rinku Kumar
63	9789355387455	Python Programming	Rupesh Nasre
64	9789355387189	Renewable Energy Technologies	Sanjay Agrawal, Rajeev K. Mishra
65	9789355387479	Software Engineering	Salman Abdul Moiz
66	9789355389749	Theory of Machines & Mechanisms	G. C. Mohan Kumar
67	9789355387332	Theory of Structures	Arunachalam Subramanian Balu
68	9789355389015	Thermal Engineering - I	V. Raghavan
69	9789355389831	Thermal Engineering - II	Parvesh Antil
70	9789355386779	Transportation Engineering (Theory & Practice)	A.K. Raji, K.K. Babu
71	9789355384287	Water Resource Engineering (Theory & Practice)	Prakash C. Swain, Dillip K. Ghose
72	9789355383051	Web Technologies: Theory & Practical	Raman Dugyala

- **Step 3:** In this step, the bacteria form water in transferred into lactose or agar slant cultural media for 24 hours to 48 hours incubated at 37°C. If gas is visible after the prescribed time further detail studied are carried out to find the exact bacteria. If positive results this water is not fit for drinking and has to be treated before supplying B-coli index number for drinking water cannot be more than 10 but in generally it should be kept less than 3.

1.4.6 MPN

MPN stands for the most probable number. This is used to determine the bacteria density by using statistical methods in a given set of test tubes. MPN Index per 100 ml for various combination of test tube is given in the table. The positive test tubes are counted for a particular set and value is seen in the table against that set. This will give the most probable number of bacteria that can occur in the 100 ml water sample.

1.4.7 SAMPLING OF WATER

The water sample which is to be collected for testing of physical, chemical and bacteriological parameters with great cares. Sampling should be done with care as the test result is depends on the sampling of water. The following measures should be taken care of while doing sampling water:

- Water bottles which have to be used for sampling should be washed with dilute nitric acid and has to be sterilized.
- Care should be taken so that the inside of the bottle gets contacted only with a sample to be collated. Sample has to be taken below the surface water so that impurities of surface are not come in contact.
- While collecting water samples from underground sources. The water should be collected after pumping some amount of water.
- After collecting water samples, the proper mention of samples is to be done carefully.
- For bacteriological parameters the collected samples are to be stored in an icebox at 4°C.
- The test should start as soon as the water sample reaches the laboratory. All the bacteriological parameters are to be done within 72 hours.

1.4.8 WATER QUALITY STANDARD AS PER IS 10500

Table 1.10 shows various water quality standards give in IS code 10500:2012 for drinking water. In this table, the physical and chemical parameters are given with their acceptance limit and the permissible limit if there are no alternate sources of water. For drinking purposes the water supply scheme should not have physical or chemical parameters above the permissible limit. All units are in mg/l except for pH and color. A complete list of IS code 10500:2012 has been given in the barcode mentioned below.

Table 1.10: Water quality standards as per IS 10500:2012

S. No	Parameters	Acceptance limit	Permissible limit
1	Color	5	15
2	pH	6.5-8.5	No relaxation
3	Turbidity	1	5
4	TDS	500	2000
5	Chloride	250	1000
6	Fluoride	1	1.5
7	Boron	0.5	1
8	Calcium	75	200
9	Silver	0.1	No relaxation
10	Copper	0.05	1.5
11	Iron	0.3	No relaxation
12	Magnesium	30	100
13	Zinc	5	15
14	Total hardness	200	600
15	Aluminum	0.03	0.2
16	Free residual chlorine	0.2	1
17	Lead	0.01	No relaxation
18	Nickel	0.02	No relaxation

UNIT SUMMARY

- Different components of the water supply scheme are discussed
- Surface water sources for water supply are lakes, rivers and reservoir
- Sub-surface water sources for water supply are springs, wells, infiltration galleries, infiltration wells
- Different intake structures are discussed in detail they are river intake, canal intake, reservoir intake, and lake intake
- Demand for water supply scheme is affected by climate, city population, water quality, and type of people in the city
- Different methods for population forecasting are arithmetical increase method, geometrical increase method, incremental increase method, growth analysis method, graphical method, comparative graphic method, zonal method
- Different types of water demand for a city are domestic purposes, commercial and industrial, public use, firefighting
- Different formulas to calculate firefighting demands are Kuchling formula, John Ripley Freeman formula, Boston formula, and the National Board of Fire underwriter's formula
- Physical characteristics of water supply are taste, temperature, odor, color, turbidity

- Chemical characteristics are TDS, fluoride, chlorides, dissolved oxygen
- Different forms of nitrogen in water are discussed
- Biological characteristics such as E-coli, and B-coli index are discussed
- Water quality standards as per IS code 10500:2012 limit are given.

EXERCISE

Multiple Choice Questions

1. The firefighting demand of a city can be calculated by
   (a) Kuchling formula (b) Boston Formula
   (c) John Ripley Formula (d) All of the above
2. Which one is the components of water supply scheme
   (a) Surface water (b) Sub-surface water
   (c) Intake structures (d) ionization of water
3. Which of the following is an intake structure
   (a) River (b) Dam
   (c) Channel (d) weirs
4. Kjedhanl Nitrogen is
   (a) Ammonia nitrogen (b) Organic nitrogen
   (c) Combine both (a) and (b) (d) none of these
5. Peak factor for water demand for population more than 2 lakhs is
   (a) 2.0 (b) 1.5
   (c) 3.0 (d) 2.5
6. Design periods (in years) for water works unit is
   (a) 50 (b) 15
   (c) 20 (d) 30
7. As per IS 1172-1993 water demand per person per day for a city
   (a) 145 (b) 175
   (c) 135 (d) 200
8. Which standard is used for comparison in color parameter
   (a) silver cobalt (b) sodium cobalt
   (c) platinum cobalt (d) potassium cobalt
9. Which are the factors affecting water demand of a city
   (a) climate (b) Size of the city
   (c) water quality (d) all of the above
10. What is the acceptance limit for TDS (in mg/l)
    (a) 200 (b) 500
    (c) 2000 (d) 1000

Answer for multiply choice questions

1. **(d)**, 2. **(c)**, 3. **(a)**, 4. **(c)**, 5. **(d)**, 6. **(b)**, 7. **(c)**, 8. **(c)**, 9. **(d)**, 10. **(a)**

Short and Long Answer Type Questions

1. Write the factors which affect the water demand of a city.
2. What is firefighting demand? Write different types of firefighting demand.
3. The following decades of population of a city are 1991 years – 55000

   2001 years – 67000

   2011 years – 81000

   2021 years – 98000

   Find population in year 2031 and 2041 using arithmetical method and geometrical method
4. What is an infiltration gallery? Explain its uses
5. Differentiate between infiltration wells and tube wells.
6. What is a pH value?
7. Explain procedure to identify E-coli in water sample.
8. Differentiate between river intake and Lake Intake.
9. Why bacteriological characteristic important for water supply scheme.
10. Write different types of chemical parameters for water supply.

REFERENCES AND SUGGESTED READINGS

1. Garg, S.K., Environmental Engineering Vol. I and Vol. II, Khanna Publishers
2. Sharma S.C, Environmental Engineering, Khanna Publishing House, New Delhi
3. Punmia, B C, Environmental Engineering, vol. I and II, Laxmi Publishers
4. Basak N N, Environmental Engineering, McGraw Hill Publishers.
5. Is code 1172-1993 (reaffirmed 2007)
6. IS code 10500:2012
7. Manual on water supply and treatment system, MOHUA, Government of India (2023)
8. Bardsley DA. B. coli as an Index of Faecal Pollution of Water Supplies. J Hyg (Lond). 1926 Feb;25(1):11-25. doi: 10.1017/s0022172400017186.

2 Purification of Water

UNIT SPECIFICS

Through this unit we have discussed the following aspects:

- *To understand various purification process involved in water treatment*
- *Process of sedimentation and coagulation*
- *Different types of filtration process*
- *Overview of disinfection and chlorination*
- *Discussion on defluoridation techniques*
- *Introduction of water softening*

To help the students in the visualization of the content and to enhance their practical knowledge, the figures are provided in 2D. The content in this unit offers practical knowledge and will help the students in decision-making during the fieldwork.

This unit contains short and long answer-type questions along with multiple choice questions, a list of references, and suggested reading so that one can go through them for practice. Some QR codes are given which can be scanned for more information on various topics of interest and to get extra knowledge.

RATIONALE

This unit on the purification of water helps the students to develop an idea about the layout of the water treatment plants. It explains the process of the purification of water. The various treatment units used for the purification are discussed. A brief discussion of the sedimentation and their types is provided. The various filtration methods are also discussed and an introduction about the water softening is given. The content covered in this unit is important to understand the process of purification of water.

The knowledge of various units of water purification and their components is essential for civil engineering students. The students can apply the knowledge of the purification of water during designing water treatment plants. The knowledge gained in this unit will help the students to identify suitable units for different types of raw water. The students can apply their knowledge in the selection and implementation of suitable defluoridation techniques during the treatment process. The concepts in this unit will help the student in effective supervision of working of water treatment plants.

PRE-REQUISITES

A basic knowledge of water properties is required.

UNIT OUTCOMES

The list of outcomes of this unit is as follows:

U2-O1: *To explain the process of the aeration.*

U2-O2: *To understand the process of sedimentation and sedimentation with coagulation.*

U2-O3: *To realize the suitability of different filtration process.*

U2-O4: *To determine the function and suitability of different types of chlorination.*

U2-O5: *To propose a suitable purification techniques method for water treatment.*

Unit-2 Outcomes	EXPECTED MAPPING WITH COURSE OUTCOMES (1- Weak Correlation; 2- Medium correlation; 3- Strong Correlation)				
	CO-1	CO-2	CO-3	CO-4	CO-5
U2-O1	-	1	-	2	-
U2-O2	-	1	-	2	-
U2-O3	-	1	-	2	-
U2-O4	-	1	-	2	-
U2-O5	1	-	-	3	-

2.1 Introduction

In the previous unit, you got the idea of where the water is collected for water treatment units and different methods of population forecasting. The water that is collected from the surface and subsurface is treated before supplying to industrial, domestic, and public use. The treatment required for a particular source depends on the physical, chemical, and biological characteristics of water, quantity, and quality of water required for use. The available water should be purified in such a way that it can be used for domestic as well as industrial uses. Various purification methods are available which depend on the quality of raw water and the quality of water required for supply.

2.2 Objective of water treatment

Raw water which is supplied after the water treatment unit is known as 'treated water'. Water treatment is mainly done to make water free from various impurities. The main objectives of the water treatment are

- Water after treatment should be free from color, odor, and taste.
- Removal of minerals from hard water to prevent the scaling of boiler and stains from clothes.
- Dissolved, suspended and colloidal impurities from raw water are to be removed by water treatment
- A different dissolved gas that is objectionable in water has to be removed.
- After treatment water should be suitable for domestic and industrial use.
- Pathogenic bacteria should be completely removed from water and it should remain free till they reach the consumer.

2.3 Aeration

2.3.1 Objects

In the aeration process, excessive air is added to water. In this process, the water comes in contact with air, it causes increase in dissolved oxygen concentration and removal of carbon dioxide and other dissolved gases from raw water, with the process of oxidation. With this process, the iron and manganese are removed to some extent from raw water. With the help of aeration some pathogenic bacteria are also removed. The smell of water due to hydrogen sulfide is removed with the aeration process. These processes help in overall improvement in the physical, chemical, and biological characteristics of raw water.

2.3.2 Methods of Aeration

Different methods of aeration in the water treatment process are:

i. Spray nozzle method
ii. Cascade method
iii. Diffusion of air method
iv. Trickling bed method

1. Spray nozzle method: In this method, the water comes in contact with air by spraying water in the atmosphere through the nozzle with a pressure which breaks water into fine droplets thus helping in releasing the dissolved gases. Contaminated gas such as carbon dioxide is removed up to 90 % through this process. This method requires a high head as water has to be sprayed into the atmosphere. A head of 10 to 15 m is required for proper working of this method. Figure 2.1 shows the spray nozzle method.

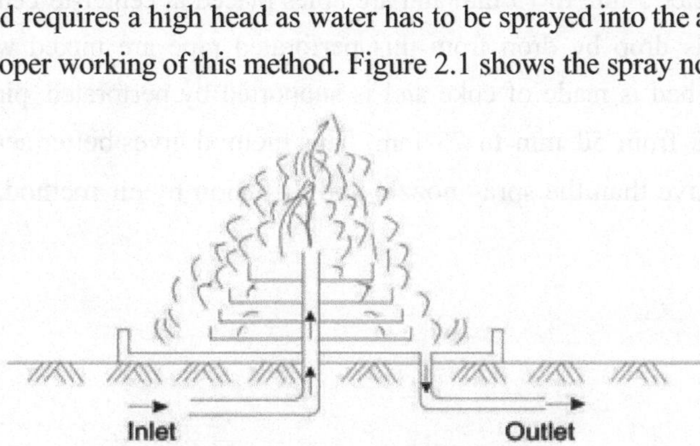

Figure 2.1: Spray Nozzle Method

2. Cascade method: In the cascade method, the water falls under gravity from a height of 2 to 3 m on a series of four to ten steps with each step having a height of 150 cm to 300 cm. The steps are made of natural stones or concrete. Figure 2.2 shows the cascade aeration. These types of structures are installed in the open air. In this method when water falls on steps it comes in contact with free air which in turn helps in increasing the concentration of dissolved oxygen. This method is less efficient than the spray method for reducing carbon dioxide gas in water. In this method up to 60 % to 70 % of carbon dioxide gas is removed. Natural waterfall and weirs is a type of natural cascade aeration.

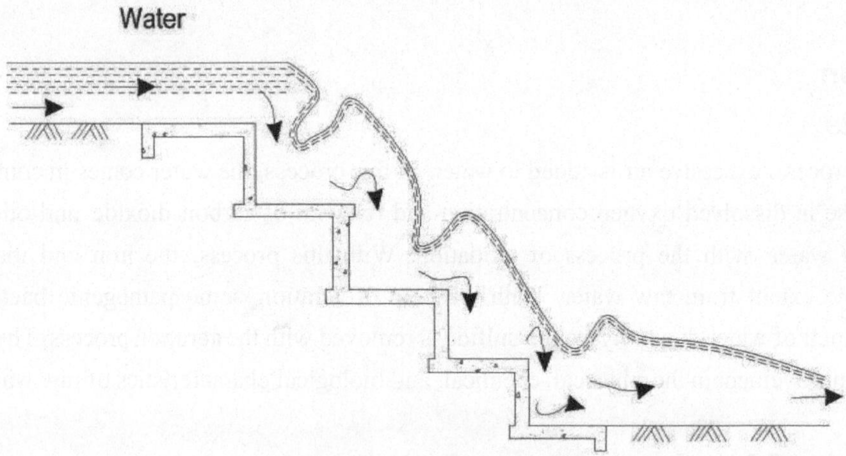

Figure 2.2: Cascade Method

3. Diffusion of air method: In this method, the air is diffused into the water using perforated pipes, so that it gets completely mixed with the water. The perforated pipes are installed at the bottom of the sedimentation tank and compressed air is sent through these pipes. When compressed air moves from the bottom of the tank to the upward direction it gets completely mixed with the water, thus completing the aeration process. In this method, air gets more time to mix in water and better aeration of water takes place compared to the cascade and spray nozzle methods.

4. Trickling bed method: In this method, water is moved down from perforated pipes. The perforated pipes have holes of diameter 5 mm to 15 mm and are holes placed at center-to-center distances of 25 mm to 75 mm. The waterfalls drop by drop from this perforated pipe are mixed with air and aeration is completed. The trickling bed is made of coke and is supported by perforated pipes. The size of coke gravels to be used varies from 50 mm to 75 mm. This method gives better aeration than the cascade method but is less effective than the spray nozzle and diffusion by air method. Figure 2.3 shows the trickling bed.

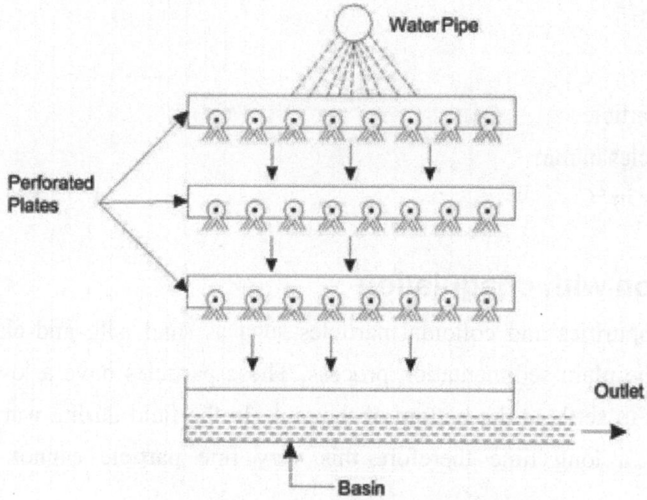

Figure 2.3: Trickling Bed Aeration

The aeration process helps remove iron, magnesium, and volatile gas. Carbon dioxide is not completely removed by the aeration process a residual of 3 mg/l to 5 mg/l is always left. Residual oil, vegetation, and algae are removed by aeration from water, which helps remove color, odor, and taste. If aeration is not used in controlled ways it will make the water corrosive which in turn necessitates the de-aeration process.

2.4 Plain Sedimentation

All suspended impurities having a specific gravity greater than water will settle on the bottom of the tank due to gravitational force which should be more than the frictional resistance of the water known as drag force. When this gravitational force is more than the drag force the particles settle at the bottom with constant velocity known as settling velocity. The spherical particle settling velocity follows Stoke's law.

2.4.1 Principle of Sedimentation

This above-mentioned process in water can only be possible if there is no turbulence in the water. There are a few factors that affect the settling velocity of the water.

1. Horizontal velocity of particle which helps the particle not to settle at the bottom of the tank.
2. Shape and size of the particles
3. Viscosity of the water

Stokes law equation 2.1 and equation 2.2 for different sizes of particles to calculate the settling velocity re given below:

a) Particle diameter up to 0.1 mm $v_s = 418(G-1)d^2\left[\frac{3T+70}{100}\right]$ ...2.1

b) Particle diameter from 0.1 mm to 1.0 mm $v_s = 418(G-1)d\left[\frac{3T+70}{100}\right]$ ...2.2

Where,

v_s = Settling velocity

G = Specific density of particle

d = Diameter of the particles in mm

T = temperature of water in °C

2.4.2 Sedimentation with coagulation

Very fine suspended impurities and colloidal particles such as sand, silt, and clay do not settle at the bottom of the tank in the plain sedimentation process. These particles have a low settling value due to which they several days to settle at the bottom of the tank. In the field during water treatment we cannot collect water for such a long time therefore this very fine particle cannot be removed in plain sedimentation.

These particles can be removed by increasing their size and changing into flocculated particles. For making flocculated particles certain chemical compounds are added in water. These chemicals are known as coagulants. When they are added in water small floc are formed and very fine suspended and colloidal particles are attached to this floc and formed bigger flocculated particles. These flocculated particles having higher specific gravity than water settle at the bottom of the tank. Sedimentation with coagulation is necessary when water has a turbidity of more than 30 to 40 mg/l.

The entire process of chemical addition and formation of flocculated particles is known as coagulation. This coagulation water is then passed through a sedimentation tank for the removal of flocculated particles.

2.4.3 Principles of coagulation

Colloidal particles having surface charges result in the adsorption and ionization of chemical compounds on the colloidal particle surface. Most colloidal particles in water are negatively charged. The charged surface is surrounded by the bound or rigid layer of water known as the stern layer as shown in figure 2.4. In the stern layer, the particle having an opposite charge in nature drawn from water towards colloidal particle and thus drops the potential known as stern potential. After the stern layer further drop in potential occur which is known as zeta potential which occurs between the shear surfaces of bound of water to the point where surface neutrality occurs in the water as shown in figure 2.4.

The charges on the surface of colloidal particles give more stability and hence it repels the like charge particles due to which they do not settle. So, coagulation is a technique in which colloidal particles are neutralized whereas in flocculation these neutralized particles are agglomerated due to slow mixing.

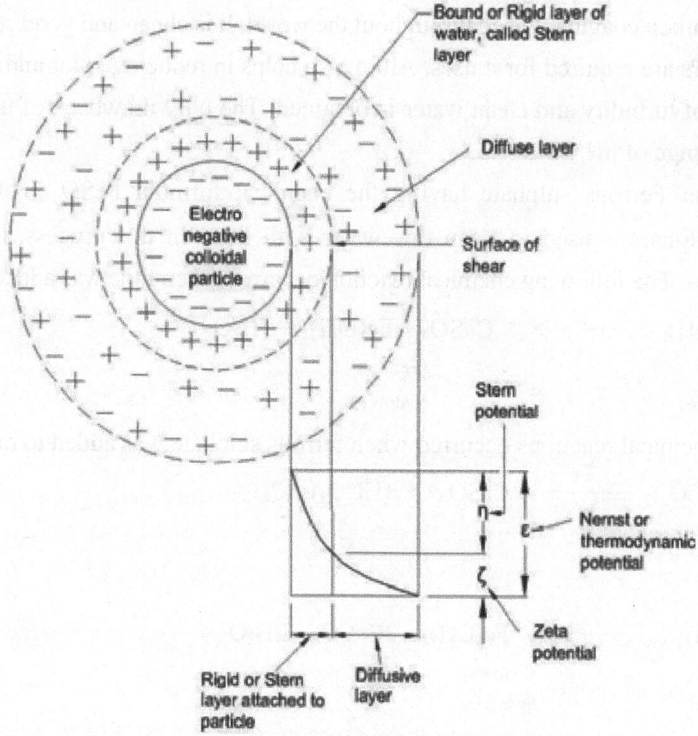

Figure 2.4: Colloidal particles

2.4.4 Types of coagulants

Different types of coagulants are available in markets based on iron or aluminum metals and can be used alone or in combination with other available coagulants. The chemicals used as coagulants in water are most effective when the water is slightly alkaline. If raw water is not alkaline then an external alkaline source such as sodium carbonate or calcium oxide is added in water to make it alkaline. Various coagulants are discussed below:

1. Alum: Aluminium sulphate ($Al_2(SO_4)_3.18H_2O$) is known as alum. When it is mixed with raw water it reacts with the alkalinity of bicarbonate ions and forms a precipitate of aluminum hydroxide. These flocs attract the colloidal particles and fine suspended particles and grow in size which ultimately settle at the bottom of the tank.

$$Al_2(SO_4)_3.18H_2O + 3Ca(HCO_3)_2 \longrightarrow 3CaSO_4 + 2Al(OH)_3(ppt.) + 6CO_2\ (gas)$$

The above chemical reaction shows how the aluminum hydroxide precipitate formed in water. In the above reaction, it can be seen that by adding the alum the permanent hardness of the water in the form of calcium sulphate is increased.

The dose of alum for the formation of flocs in raw water depends on the turbidity and color. The optimum dose of alum can be calculated in the laboratory on the batch scale and the same result can be implemented in the treatment plant. The dose of alum varies from 5 mg/l to 85 mg/l depending on the turbidity of water. The average dose of alum is 17 mg/l.

Alum is the most common coagulant used throughout the world. It is cheap and good stable flocs are formed and no skilled workers are required for it uses. Alum also helps in reducing color and improves the taste in addition to removal of turbidity and clean water is obtained. The only drawback of using alum is that it is effective in a small range of pH 6.5 to 8.3.

2. Ferrous sulphate: Ferrous sulphate having the chemical formula $FeSO_4.7H_2O$ is also known as copperas. Ferrous sulphate is used to clean raw water with lime. In this process, lime can be added to copperas or vice-versa. The following chemical reaction occurred when lime was added before copperas.

$$FeSO_4.7H_2O + Ca(OH)_2 \longrightarrow CaSO_4 + Fe(OH)_2 + 7H_2O$$

(Lime Hydrated) (Ferrous hydroxide)

The following two chemical reactions occurred when ferrous sulphate was added to raw water before lime.

$$FeSO_4.7H_2O + Ca(HCO_3)_2 \longrightarrow CaSO_4 + Fe(HCO_3)_2 + 7H_2O$$

(Alkalinity in raw water)

$$Fe(HCO_3)_2 + 2Ca(OH)_2 \longrightarrow Fe(OH)_2 + 2CaCO_3 + 2H_2O$$

(Lime Hydrated) (Ferrous hydroxide)

In above mention both cases ferrous hydroxide formed is further oxidized in water to form ferric hydroxide. The chemical reaction is given below:

$4Fe(OH)_2 + O_2 + 2H_2O \longrightarrow 4Fe(OH)_3$ (Ferric hydroxide precipitate) The ferric hydroxide precipitate formed helps in the removal of colloidal particles.

Ferrous sulphate is a coagulant used to treat the raw water which is not colored. It is relatively cheaper than alum and can be used to treat raw water having a pH greater than 8.5. The amount of ferrous sulphate used to treat raw water is the same as that of alum.

3. Chlorinated Copperas: In this process, chlorine is added to ferrous sulphate solution and they chemically react due to which the formation of ferric sulphate and ferric chloride take place. The reaction that occurred is given below.

$$6(FeSO_4.7H_2O) + 3Cl_2 \longrightarrow 2Fe_2(SO_4)_3 + 2FeCl_3 + 42H_2O$$

The combination of ferric sulphate and ferric chloride is known as chlorinated copperas. It is used to treat raw water colored and it can also be used in places where the raw water has a low pH. Ferric sulfate when used with hydrated lime formed flocs of ferric hydroxide which in turn helps in the removal of colloidal particles.

When raw water has pH range of 4 to 7 and pH above 9 ferric sulphate gives quite a good result whereas in the case of ferric chloride the range of pH should be 3.5 to 6.5 and pH above 8.5 is good. Therefore as we can see this combination is quite useful for treating raw water with low pH value.

4. Sodium Aluminate: The chemical formula of sodium aluminate is $Na_2Al_2O_4$. Sometimes this can be used as a coagulant in place of alum and iron based coagulants. Sodium aluminate when used as a coagulant mixed with raw water reacts with calcium and magnesium salts present in water to for the precipitate of calcium aluminate and magnesium aluminate. The various chemical reactions involved in the removal process are given below.

$$Na_2Al_2O_4 + Ca(HCO_3)_2 \longrightarrow CaAl_2O_4(ppt) + Na_2CO_3 + CO_2 + H_2O$$

$$Na_2Al_2O_4 + CaCl_2 \longrightarrow CaAl_2O_4(ppt) + 2NaCl$$

$$Na_2Al_2O_4 + CaSO_4 \longrightarrow CaAl_2O_4(ppt) + Na_2SO_4$$

Sodium aluminate is 1.5 times costly than alum so, it is not used for treating raw water for general public uses. It can be used to treat water which cannot be treated using alum for example the water which do not have alkalinity are treated with this process.

With the help of using sodium aluminate for treatment it can be seen by chemical reaction that it helps in removal of temporary as well as permanent hardness from raw water that cannot be possible in case of using alum. Raw water treated with process is used for feeding in boiler as boiler water required very low amount of hardness.

2.4.5 Jar test

Jar test is the most common test to find out the optimum coagulant dose required for the treatment plant. Figure 2.5 show the apparatus used for jar test. In these test 6 beakers of same size and 1liter capacity is taken. Six jars should have same amount of water and different amount of coagulant in each jar is added. After adding the coagulant driving unit is started. There is a paddle in each jar for mixing the coagulant properly which is connected with driving shaft through vertical rods. Paddles are rotate and floc formation in each jar is checked. The jar having good amount of floc using least amount of coagulant will indicate the optimum dose of coagulant. For knowing the least optimum dose of coagulant the paddle speed and mixing time also varied for different sets.

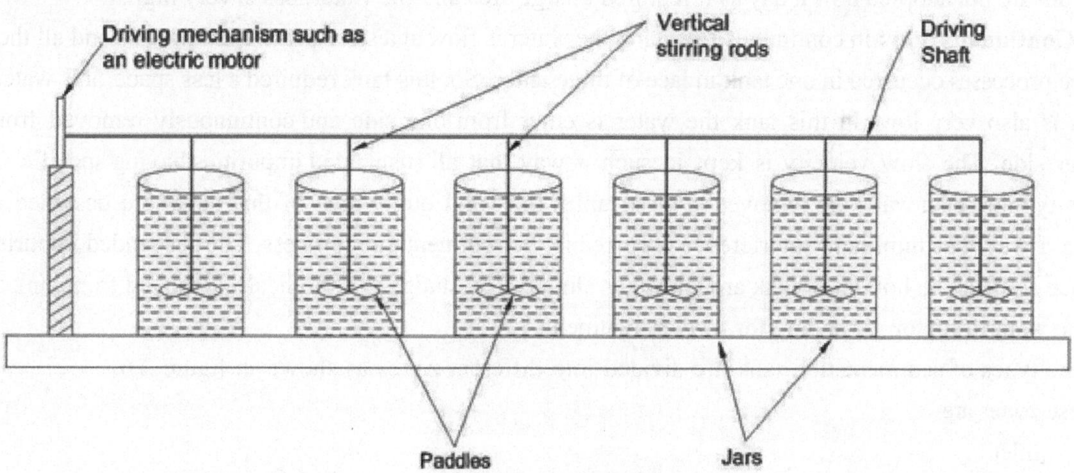

Figure 2.5: Jar Test

2.4.6 Process of coagulation

In coagulation process the first step is to feed the chemical in dry or in solution form into raw water. After feeding the thoroughly mixing of chemical take place in mixing basin. This mixing helps the coagulant to get fully dispersed into raw water. Mixing device used for mixing the water are centrifugal pumps, compressed are and mixing basins. In mixing basins there are baffle walls and mechanical devise are incorporated for proper mixing.

The chemical reactions which occur in mixing basin result in the formation of floc which is allowed to consolidate in flocculation tank. In flocculation tank the water is slow mixed to allow flocs to get agglomeration. Flocculation tank are rectangular in shape are fitted with paddle which are operated with electric motors. In this tank the paddle are rotated at 2 to 3 rpm and a detention period is kept from 20 to 60 minutes. This flocculated after slow mixing complete pass to sedimentation tank where they settle at the bottom of the tank. The complete process of coagulation helps in removing the turbidity from raw water. Coagulation also helps in removing of bacteria and help in reducing b-coli index up to 70 %.

2.4.7 Types of sedimentation tanks

Sedimentation tanks basically divided into two types based on the flow are:

(1) Intermittent flow: In intermittent tank water is allowed to remain still after filling the tank. The tank remains stable till all suspended impurities settle at the bottom of the sedimentation tank. This type of tank has a large detention period of more than 24 hours. When these detention periods over the pure water are removed. For this type of tank a large area is required as we required at least three sets of intermittent sedimentation tank for treatment plant to work smoothly. In first tank the water is filled while in second tank the sedimentation process is occurring and in third tank the water is removing after sedimentation these three process will occurring simultaneously at same time in three different tanks. These types of system are not adopted now a day as it required a large area and the water loss is very high.

(2) Continuous flow: In continuous flow tank the water is flow at a steady rate continuously and all the three processes occurred in one tank in lace of three tanks. So, this tank required a less space and water loss is also very low. In this tank the water is enter from one side and continuously removed from other side. The flow velocity is kept in such a way that all suspended impurities having specific gravity more than water are removed in these tanks. Inlet and outlet area of this tanks are designed in such a way that minimum interference occurred in the sedimentation process. The suspended impurities which settle at the bottom of tank are known as sludge. The sludge is periodically removed from tank and clean water from top is sending for further treatment.

These types of sedimentation tank are divided into different zones as shown in figure 2.6.

These zones are

a. Inlet

b. Settling

c. Sludge

d. Outlet

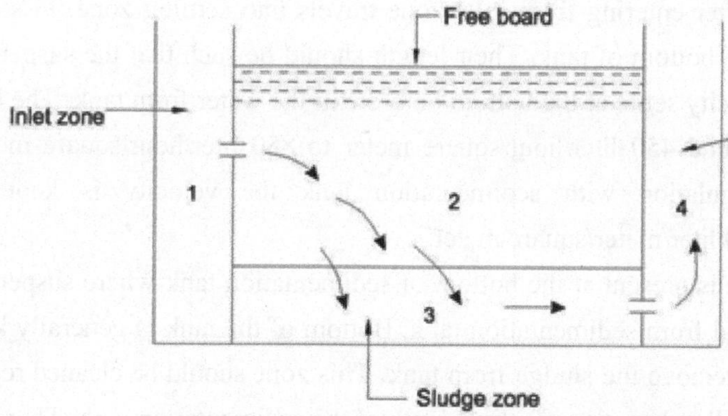

Figure 2.6: Different zones of sedimentation tank

a. **Inlet zones:** Inlet zone are setup at one side of the tank from where the water enters into the tank. This zone is created to reduce the velocity of water and to control the movement of water. In this zone a baffle wall is installed at the entry of inlet pipe. Inlet pipe in this zone are installed in such a way that entire width of tank receive equal water. If there is any disturbance at the entry of water which will affect the sedimentation process and proper settling will not occur. Figure 2.7 shows different types of inlet in sedimentation tank from where the water enters to sedimentation tank.

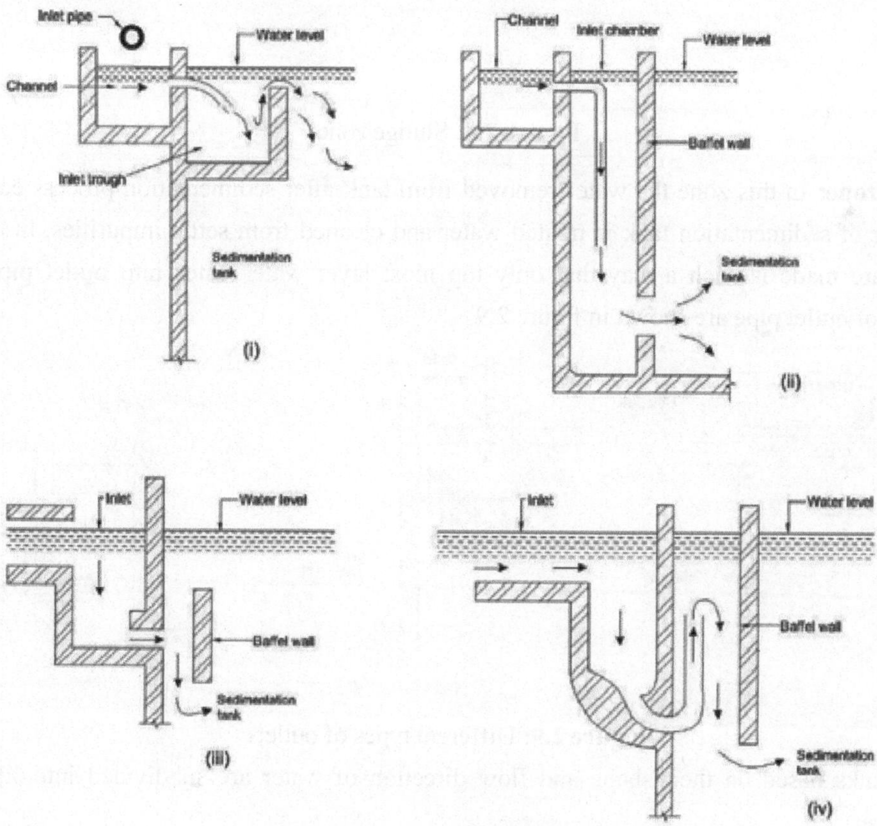

Figure 2.7: Various types of inlets

b. Settling zone: Water after entering from inlet zone travels into settling zone. In settling zone the suspended particle settle at the bottom of tank. Their length should be such that the suspended impurities following horizontal flow velocity settle at the bottom before exit the water from tank. The horizontal flow velocity is generally kept around 450 liter/hour/square meter to 850 liter/hour/square meter for normal sedimentation tank. In coagulation with sedimentation tank the velocity is kept around 1000 liter/hour/square meter to 1500 liter/meter/square meter.

c. Sludge zone: This zone is present at the bottom of sedimentation tank where suspended impurities settle and collected for removal from sedimentation tank. Bottom of the tank is generally kept at slope as shown in figure 2.8 to easily remove the sludge from tank. This zone should be cleaned regularly at fixed interval of time otherwise it will reduce the effective depth of the sedimentation tank. There is value at the bottom of the tank through which sludge is removed.

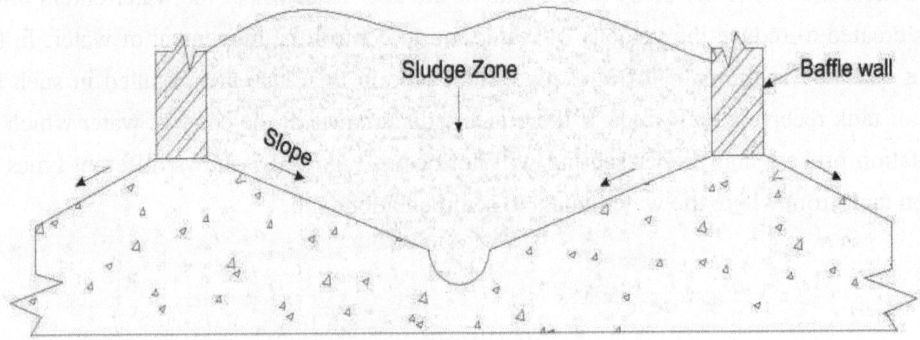

Figure 2.8: Sludge zone

d. Outlet zone: In this zone the water removed from tank after sedimentation process complete. The top most layer of sedimentation tank is treated water and cleaned from settle impurities. In this zone the arrangement are made is such a way that only top most layer water enter into outlet pipe. Different arrangements of outlet pipe are shown in figure 2.9

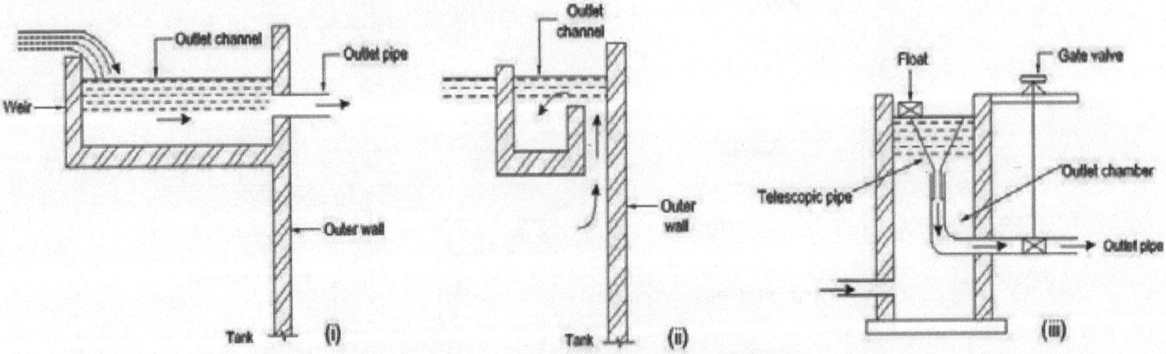

Figure 2.9: Different types of outlets

Continuous tanks based on their shape and flow direction of water are subdivided into different types. They are:

i. Rectangular tank with longitudinal flow

ii. Circular tank with redial flow

iii. Hopper bottom tank with vertical flow

The working of above mention sedimentation tanks are explained in below section.

i. **Rectangular tank with longitudinal flow:** This type of tanks is rectangular in shape having concrete base and side walls are made up of bricks works. In these tanks various baffle walls are made in the middle of tanks as shown in the figure 2.10. These baffles wall helps in increasing the flow path and helps in reducing the velocity of flowing water which in turns helps in increasing sedimentation. Bottom of the tank is sloped between two baffle walls as shown in figure 2.10.

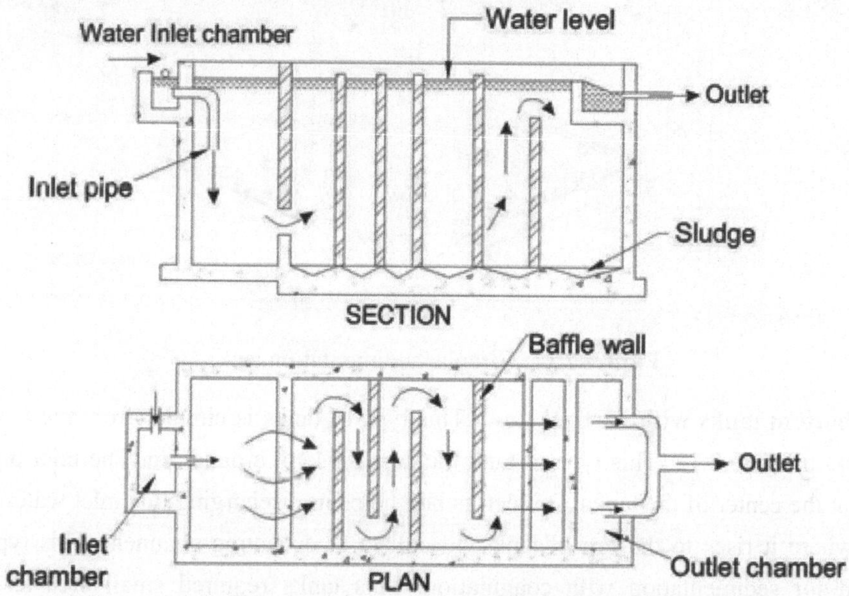

Figure 2.10: Rectangular sedimentation tank

This tanks having a length of around 50 m and there width is kept around 10 m. the depth of the tank varies from 3 m to 5 m. the detention time of the flowing water is kept around 4 hours for which the flow velocity is kept around 0.6 m/min to 0.9 m/min.

ii. **Circular sedimentation tank with radial flow:** This type of tanks having circular shape with base slope at the center. This tank do not have baffle wall and work better than the rectangular tank as particle settle same at all points. In this tank the water flows from the center of the tank to the radial direction to side of the tank. For this a vertical inlet pipe is kept at the center of the tank and outlet pipe are made at the perimeter of the tank as shown in figure 2.11 There are deflector box which helps in diverting the water coming from inlet pipe. With the help of deflector arm the water is released near the bottom of tank from where it travels to the periphery of the tank and will rising the water the suspended impurities settle at the bottom of tank.

At the bottom of the tank there are raking arms which helps in collecting the sludge. These raking arms are mechanically rotated at a slow speed. The blades in raking arms scrap the sludge from the bottom surface and helps in moving it into the sinks pit made at the center of the tank as shown in figure 2.11.

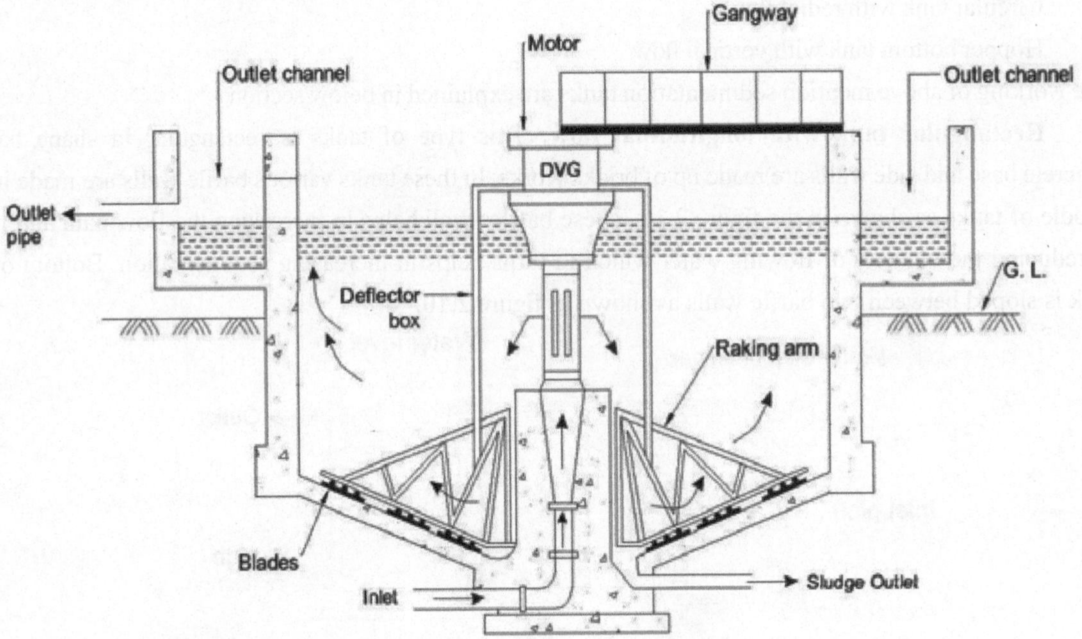

Figure 2.11: Circular sedimentation tank

iii. **Hopper bottom tanks with vertical flow:** This type of tanks is circular from the top with hopper bottom as shown in figure 2.12. This type of tank the depth is kept around 5m. The inlet pipes discharge water from top at the center of the tanks. Deflectors box helps in discharging this inlet water at the bottom of tanks from where it rises to the top of tank and collect at decanting channels. This type of tanks is generally suited for sedimentation with coagulation. This tanks required small area as compared to rectangular tanks. Vertical flow tanks are better as compared to horizontal flows but there construction is costly.

2.4.8 Clariflocculator

Clariflocculator is a single circular tanks made up of two concentric tanks in which the outer tanks act as clarifier while inner tanks flocculation process occur as shown in figure 2.13. In this tank water from inlet pipes enter to inner flocculation tank where the water is gently mixed with the help of paddles to form the flocs. These flocs moves to the peripheral of the tank to clarifier tanks where the flocs are settle at the bottom of the tanks and clean water from top surface discharge for further treatment.

The detention time in this tank is kept 10 minute to 40 minutes with inlet flow velocity of around 0.2 m/sec to 0.8 m/sec. depth of the tank is vary from 2.5 m to 5 m. The paddle revolves at 1 to 2 rpm.

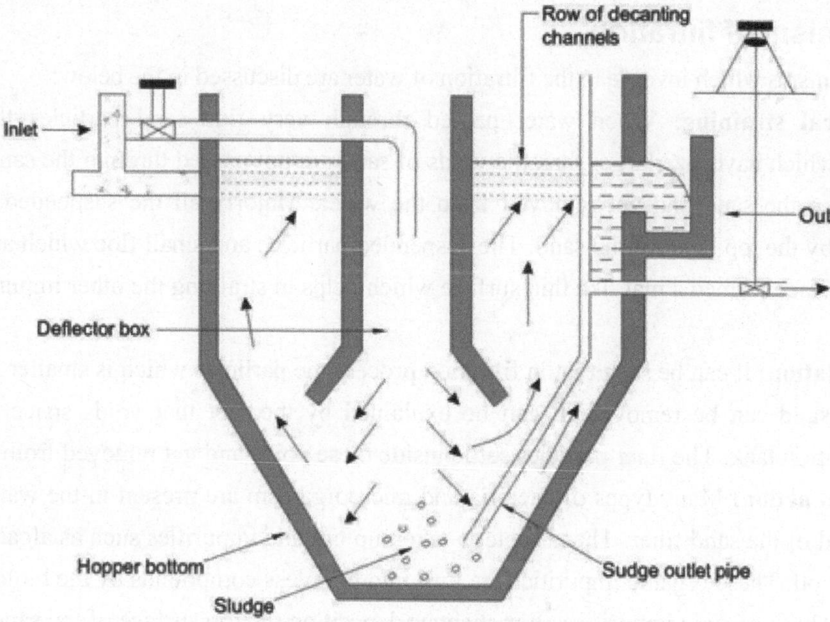

Figure 2.12: Hopper bottom tanks

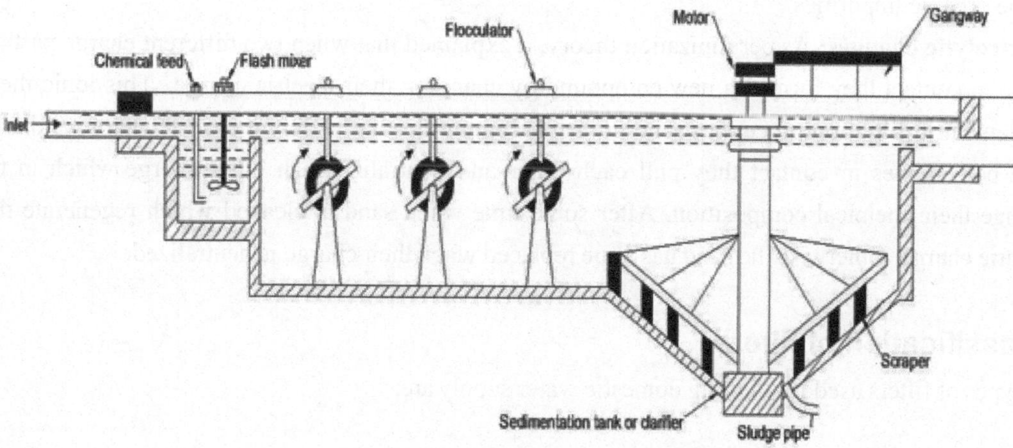

Figure 2.13: Clarifloccculator

2.5 Filtration

In sedimentation process a huge percentage of suspended impurities are removed from raw water. While using coagulation with sedimentation very fine colloidal particles are also easily removed. But after sedimentation process a very fine discrete particle, small flocs after coagulation and bacteria in water is still remained. To make water free from this impurities and drinkable it is further filtered by passing through fine sand particles. The process in which water is passed through several layer of very fine sand and granular materials is known as filtration. In this process color, taste, odor, turbidity and bacteria are removed from water.

2.5.1 Mechanism of filtration

Different mechanisms which involve in the filtration of water are discussed in the below:

(1) **Mechanical straining:** When water passed through very fine sand particles then suspended particles which have size larger than the voids of sand are not passed through the sand filter and are retained on the sand and get removed from the water. Majorly all the suspended impurities are removed by the top layer of the sand. The suspended particles and small floc which are remained on the top surface formed a mat like thin surface which helps in straining the other impurities present in water.

(2) **Sedimentation:** It can be seen that in filtration process the particles which is smaller in size then the voids of sand can be removed. It can be explained by the fact that voids space in sand act as sedimentation tank. The finer particles settle inside these voids and get removed from water.

(3) **Biological action:** Many types of bacteria and microorganism are present in the water are attached to the void of the sand filter. These bacteria taken up organic impurities such as algae, plankton etc. as there food. These organic impurities are turn into harmless compounds by the biological action of bacteria. These organic impurities after changes deposit on the top surface of the sand and formed a gelatin film known as schmutzdecke. This gelatin film layer helps in further staining and absorbing of the organic impurities.

(4) **Electrolytic changes:** As per ionization theory, it explained that when two different charge particles come in contact they formed a new compound by changing their electric charge. This ionic theory implement in filtration process as sand grains and impurities has different electric charge and when they both comes in contact they pull each other and neutralize each other charge which in turn change their chemical composition. After some time when sand is cleaned which regenerate their electric charge. Otherwise the sand has to be replaced when their charge is neutralized.

2.5.2 Classification of filters

Different types of filters used for treating domestic water supply are:

2.5.2.1 Slow sand filter

Slow sand filter are invented by James Simpson in England in 1829. As the name suggest in this filtration process the rate of filtration is very slow. The filtration occurs in this process due to gravitational force so they are also known as gravity filters. Their operation is very simple and used for small town or rural areas.

2.5.2.2 Construction and working of slow sand filtration

Slow sand filter has different components as shown in figure 2.14. First components are the filter tanks which are made up of concrete or brick works with top surface open. They are generally rectangular in shape with area varies from 100 m^2 to 2000 m^2. The depth of the tank is kept around 2.5 m to 3.5 m with a slope of 1:100 toward central drain line. Different layer of sand is filled in the tank. Sand layer varies from 90 cm to 110 cm with gravel support at their bottom. Effective size of the sand varies from 0.25 mm to 0.4 mm with uniform coefficient ranges from 1.80 to 2.50. Very fine layer of sand is generally kept at the top surface. Gravel support thickness is around 60 cm to 90 cm with size of gravels ranges from 6 mm to 65 mm. Under drain pipe are installed at the bottom to collect the filtered water. Perforated pipes are used for drain pipes and kept parallel to the slope and connected to the central drain pipe.

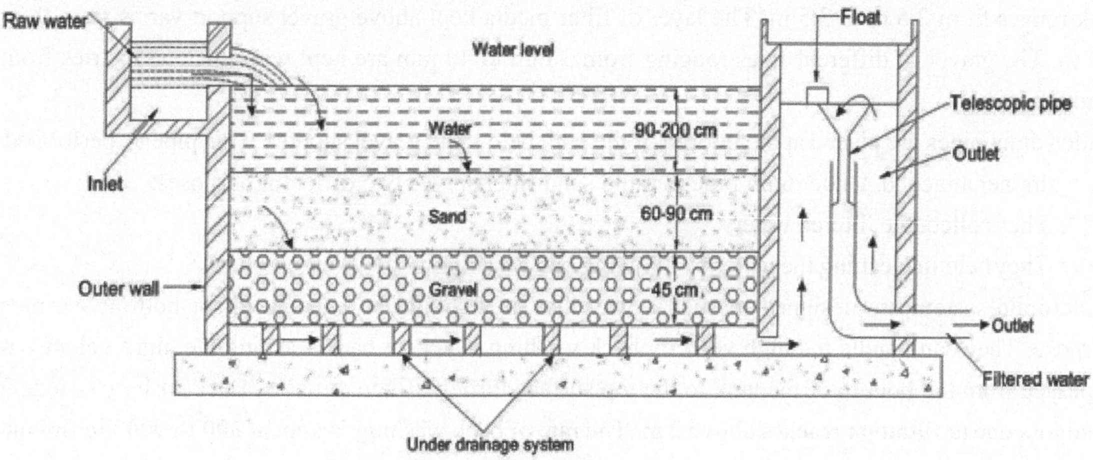

Figure 2.14: Slow Sand Filter

Treated water from the sedimentation tank is enter slowly from the top surface and passed through different layers of sand and gravels. After reaching at the bottom of gravels it enters into under drain pipes and that's leads to central drain pipe. Very fine suspended impurities and organic matter accumulate at the top surface of the filter media. Rate of filtration is generally kept constant by using telescopic tubes.

The cleaning of slow sand filter is done by removing top sand layer of 1.5 cm to 3 cm. The clean of sand require a lot labors as the top surface sand is racked, cleaned and wash with good water. The rate of filtration attained by slow sand filter is around 100 to 200 liter/hr/m^2 of filter area.

Slow sand filter removed around 98%-99% of bacterial impurities and all types of suspended impurities. This type of filter removed taste and odor caused by organic matter. They are not efficient for removing color from raw water. They can remove turbidity up to 50 mg/l. they are not recommended if raw water having high turbidity.

2.5.2.3 Rapid Sand Filter

This filter work as same as slow sand filter but they have sand particles larger than the slow sand filter so that there rate of filtration is high. This filter helps in reducing the land requirements as compared to slow sand filter. In larger and congested cities where the land is costly and water requirement is high, the rapid sand filtration is necessary as it required less area and rate of filtration is high. In this process filtration occurred due to gravitation force so they also known as rapid gravity filter.

2.5.2.4 Construction and working of rapid sand filtration

Rapid sand filters generally use coarse sand having an effective size of sand more than 0.5 mm and a uniform coefficient of sand varies from 1.3 m to 1.7 m. This filter treats 30 times more water than a slow sand filter. Sedimentation with coagulation tank water is filtered through this filtration process. The various components of the rapid sand filter are shown in figure 2.15.

The filter tank of a rapid sand filter is rectangular and made up of brickwork or concrete. The depth of the tank ranges from 2.5 m to 3.5 m. The layer of filter media kept above gravel support varies from 0.6 m to 0.9 m. The gravel of different sizes ranging from 3 mm to 40 mm are kept with thickness varies from 0.6 m to 0.9 m.

Under-drain pipes are placed at the bottom of the tank below the gravel support. This pipe is perforated and has a strainer attached. Underdrain pipe in rapid sand filter serves two different purposes:

I. They collect the filtered water

II. They help in cleaning the water by allowing backwashing

Underdrain system are designed in such a way that they should be capable in for both above mention purpose. They can handle the high velocity back washing water. In back washing the high- velocity water is passed from the bottom of the tank to the top surface through filtered media. Backwashing is done when head loss due to filtration reaches above 2 m. The rate of back washing is kept at 300 to 900 liter/minute/m^2 of filter area. This value depends on the design in such a way that uniform distribution of water occur in gravel and sand beds. Manifold and lateral systems of under-drain pipes are used in India. Figure 2.15 Show the plan of the manifold and lateral system underdrain pipes. Pipes are installed at a distance of 0.15 m to 0.3 m apart. The central drain pipe has a diameter of 0.4 cm while the lateral pipes have a diameter of 0.1 m.

The workings of the rapid sand filter concerning (figure 2.15) are explained below. Various type of valves is used to control the flow in the tank and backwash the sand. In the first step the valve A is open from where the water from the sedimentation-coagulation tank is entered. This water filtered through coarse sand bed and collected through perforated lateral pipes at the bottom and collected by open the valve D. When water filtration process occur only this two valve are open and other are closed.

When the sand being clogged and head loss increase the filter sand has to be cleaned and washed. In backwashing process the valve A and valve D is closed and valve B and valve C and compressed air valve is opened. The compressed air and backwash water from valve C entered through the bottom of the tank and wash water was collected through valve B. The process of backwashing takes about 3 to 5 minutes. After backwashing valve C, Valve D, and the compressed air valve remained closed, and starting a few minutes the raw water after filtration passed through valve B to collect the dirty water. After that valve B is closed and Valve D is opened for normal function. The amount of water used for backwashing is about 2% to 3% of the total water filter.

Rapid sand filters as compared to slow sand filters are less efficient in removing turbidity and bacteria from water. About 80 % of bacteria were removed through a rapid sand filter. A disinfection unit is required in case of a rapid sand filter. Turbidity of water brings down to 35 mg/l to 45 mg/l. They are efficient in removing color from water.

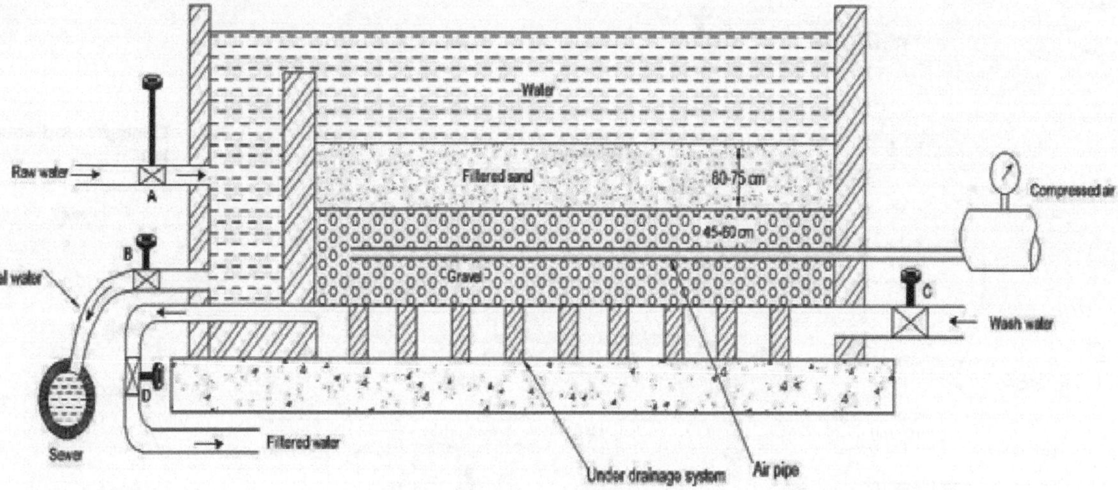

Figure 2.15: Rapid sand filter

2.5.2.5 Pressure Filter

Pressure filter are like small rapid sand filter which is placed inside the closed vessel and operate under high pressure. In this filtration process water is treated under pressure. As the pressure is higher than the atmospheric pressure this filtration requires an air-tight closed vessel. The water passed into this vessel through the help of a pump. The pressure kept in this vessel range from 300 KN/m^2 to 700 KN/m^2.

The pressure vessel can be installed in a vertical or horizontal position. In case of vertical vessel the diameter is small as compared to horizontal vessel. The diameter of vessel varies from 1.3 m to 3 m. Figure 2.16 shows the pressure filter with the horizontal vessel. The length of the pressure vessel ranges from 3.5 m to 8.5 m. Different types of valves with their position are shown in figure 2.16.

This filtration has a very high rate of filtration as water is under high pressure. This filter clogged due to high rate of filtration and often cleans in less than 24 hour of operation. The cleaning process is the same as the rapid sand filter. The rate of filtration ranges from 6000 to 15000 liter/hour/m^2 of filter area. This rate is about 2 to 5 times of a rapid sand filter.

2.5.2.6 Operational Problems in Filtration

The different problems that occurred during the operation of the filtration process are discussed below:

- **Air Binding:** when the filtration starts the initial head, loss is very small as time passes this head loss starts to increase as impurities are trapped in sand. After some time, a stage occurs when the filter resistance offered by sand particles becomes more than the static head due to water above the sand bed and due to this the negative head develops. In negative head the dissolved gas and air present in water begins to separate and formed bubble around sand bed and stick to their surface and affect the filtration process. This phenomenon is known as air bidding. To prevent the air bidding the head losses in the filtration do not increase more than 1.25 m.

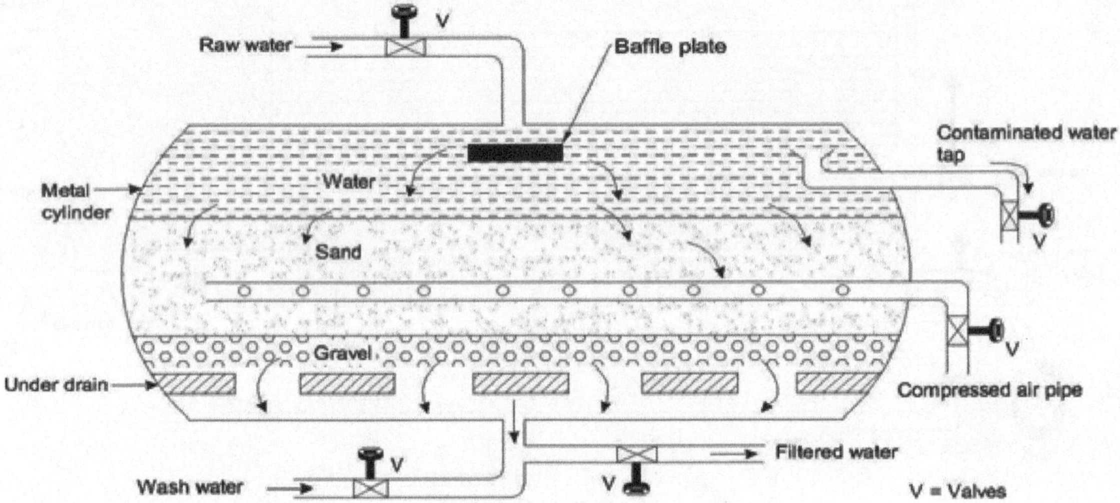

Figure 2.16: Pressure filter

- **Mud balls formation:** in the filtration process the mud from raw water get deposited on the surface of sand. During back washing process inadequate amount of water is used the sand is not washed properly this mud does not separate from the sand and sticks around the sand forming mud balls. This mud ball with time increases in size and interface in the filtration process. These mud balls are broken mechanically by using mechanical rakes or long rods.
- **Cracking in filters:** The top layer of the filter contains very fine sand which gets shrinkage and develops cracks in the filter. These cracks are major developed near the wall junction. As the pressure on the sand increase due to head loss the crack get widen. It affects the filtration process. This can be done by replacing the sand.

2.6 Disinfection

The water received after slow sand filtration or rapid sand filtration contains a lot of harmful bacteria in it. This bacterium has to be destructive or killed to make water safe of domestic water supply. To kill these bacteria a chemical is used known as disinfectants and the process in which this all occur is known as disinfection.

2.6.1 Objectives of disinfection

The disinfection process is very important in the water supply scheme because if the disinfection is not done properly then harmful pathogenic bacteria can cause various diseases and this can cause epidemics in human life. Disinfection helps in killing and destroying all pathogenic bacteria and also helps in maintain water free from bacteria afterward in the water supply.

2.6.2 Methods of disinfection

The different method which is used for killing the pathogenic bacteria is described below:

(a) **Boiling of water:** Boiling for a longer time helps in destroying the bacteria in water. This method is very helpful in killing bacteria but it is not possible to boil a large amount of water as the water supply requires a huge quantity. There is another drawback is that by boiling the existing bacteria can be killed but it cannot prevent water from future contaminations. Therefore this method cannot be used for disinfecting water supply for domestic purposes. It can only be used at the house during an epidemic.

(b) **Treatment with ozone:** Ozone gas is a good disinfectant that has a pungent smell. The color of the ozone gas is pale blue. Ozone gas is an unstable form of oxygen containing three atoms of oxygen. It can be made in the laboratory and also naturally occurs in the stratosphere. In laboratory, it made by using a closed chamber in which a high electric current is passed through the air stream. As ozone gas is very in stabile it breaks down to form oxygen molecules and nascent oxygen. This nascent oxygen is a very powerful oxidizing agent which helps in killing the bacteria.

Around 2 mg/l to 3 mg/l of ozone gas is used for treating water. Residual ozone of about 0.1 mg/l is left after a contact time of 10 minutes. This residual ozone can be measured by using an ortholoidine test. The treatment of ozone is not common as it is a costly method and required a regular supply of electricity.

(c) **Treatment with excess lime:** The use of lime normally done for removal of hardness from water but when we added excess amount of lime it kill bacteria in addition of the removal of hardness. An addition of 10 to 45 mg/l of lime helps in killing about 99% to 100% of pathogenic bacteria.

These excess additions of lime affect the pH of water and make it alkaline with a pH reaching above 9.5.this method gives very good result in terms of killing the bacteria but a higher pH has to be adjusted before water is supplied. Re-carbonation is done to adjust the pH. The drawback of this method is that it can kill the bacteria at instant but cannot protect water during supply.

(d) **Treatment with Iodine and Bromine:** In the case of disinfecting water using iodine and bromine, it kills all the bacteria in a 5-minute contact time with an amount lower than 8 mg/l. There are pills available in the market which can be used for small household or industries. This method is used to treat small supplies such as swimming polls as they are expensive and have limited uses.

(e) **Treatment with ultraviolet rays:** Ultra-violet rays having wavelength ranges from 1000 to 4000 mμ. They are not visible to the naked eye. These rays are naturally found in sun rays but can be produced in the laboratory by passing an electric current through quartz bulb carrying mercury in it. Ultraviolet rays kill all types of bacteria present in water. Water which has to be disinfect using ultra violet rays should have a turbidity less than 15 mg/l and should not have any color. In this method, the water has to be moved over the quartz bulb from where the rays are generated. This method is very expensive as continuously uses electric current and cannot be used for disinfecting large-scale water supply schemes.

(f) **Treatment with Potassium Permanganate:** Potassium permanganate is a very powerful oxidizing agent used to kill bacteria. In this method, the contact time ranges from 3 to 6 hours with doses varying from 1 mg/l to 2 mg/l. when we added potassium permanganate in water the color of water turns pink it indicate that more quantity of chemical is required to complete oxidize the organic matter. The pink color will disappear when all organic matter is oxidized. This method is cheap as compared to other method but it does not guarantee for 100 % bacteria removal.

(g) **Katadyn method:** In this method silver is used as a disinfectant material. Silver ions are generating by using solid silver electrodes which is connected to a D.C. supply of 1.5 volts. The water is disinfected by passing over this silver electrode. The contact time for disinfecting due to this method ranges from 10 minutes to 3 hours depending on dose which varies from 0.05 mg/l to 0.1 mg/l. this method do not induces ant taste and odor to the water but it is very expensive to use.

2.7 Chlorination

Chlorination is generally the addition of chlorine in water for disinfection. Chlorine in different forms is added to water and globally used for disinfection. It is cheap, easily available, quickly dissolve in water and can be handle easily. It has the most important properties that it leaves residual chlorine which keep water free from germs after a long time. It has a disadvantage in that it leaves a bitter taste in water when used in large amounts.

When we add chlorine in water it forms a temporary acid known as hypochlorous acid. This hypochlorous acid is very unstable in water and further dissociates to form hypochlorite ions and hydrogen ions as shown in below mention equation.

$$Cl_2 + H_2 \rightarrow HOCL + HCl$$

$$HOCl \leftrightarrow H^+ + OCl^-$$

The above-mentioned equation is reversible and depends on the pH of water which forms will exist in a particular pH. If the pH of water is above 8 then the dissolution of hypochlorous acid will take place and hypochlorite ions will only be present in water but if pH is less than 7 then the dominant species will be hypochlorous acid. In both of these forms, the hypochlorous acid is more effective than the other form. So for treating water with chlorine its pH kept around 7.

2.7.1 Application of chlorine

Chlorine is applied in different forms in water. They are explained in the below section

(1) **Chlorine as a powder form**: Calcium hypochlorite and sodium hypochlorite are found in powder form and used to disinfect the water. Another powder form in which chlorine is available is bleaching powder. Bleaching powder contains around 30 % of chlorine and has a white color. Bleaching powder is highly unstable in nature and loses it chlorine when comes in contact with air and moisture. It can be used for treating small quantities such as swimming pools. Around 3.0 kg of bleaching powder is sufficient for treating one million liters of water.

(2) **Chlorine as a solution form:** Chlorine in liquid form is made by dissolving chlorine gas in water. The color of liquid chlorine is amber and it is 1.5 times heavier than water. A chlorinator is a device used for adding chlorine to water. Contact time is kept around 20 to 30 minutes. Figure 2.17 shows the device used to add liquid chlorine with water known as chlorinator.

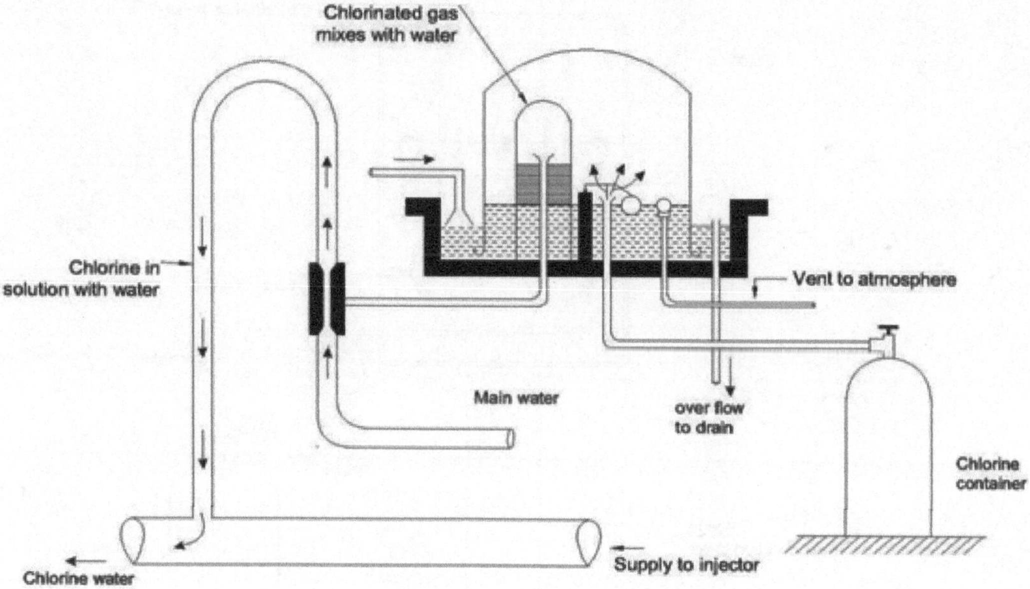

Figure 2.17: Chlorinator

(3) **Chlorine as a gas form:** Chlorine can be added directly into the water in the gaseous form. The color of chlorine gas is greenish-yellow. It is 2.5 times heavier than air. It is an inexpensive method. In this method, there is a possibility of corrosion of pipes as it gases do not completely dissolved. If the water pressure is higher than 2 kg/cm^2 it becomes difficult to dissolve chlorine gas in water. A gas chlorinator is used to mix gas in water. The chlorine gas is transported using a steel cylinder. Figure 2.18 shown the device by which gases chlorine added to water.

2.7.2 Forms of chlorination

Chlorine is available in different forms. They are

- Liquid chlorine
- Gaseous chlorine
- Chlorine dioxide
- Chloramines
- Bleaching powder

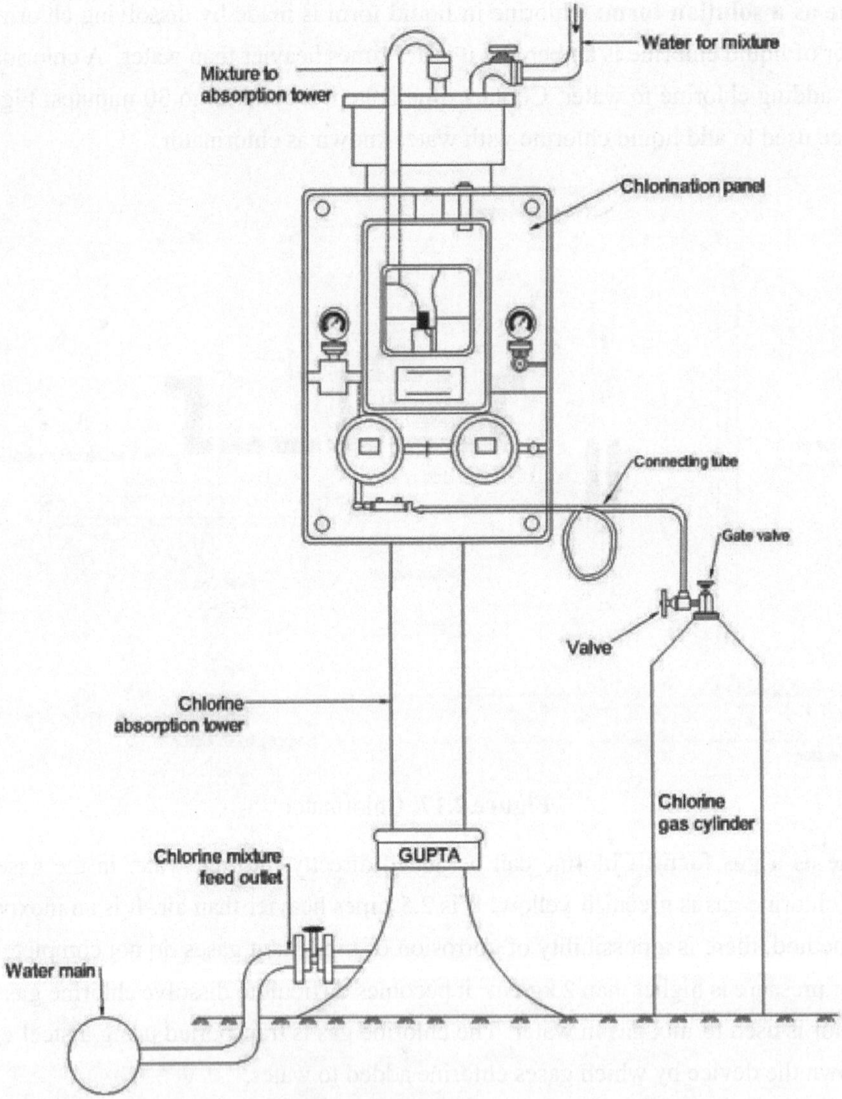

Figure 2.18: Gas chlorinator

2.7.3 Types of chlorination practice

Chlorination depends on the amount of chlorine to be added and at which stage of treatment it has to be added. Different types of chlorination practices adopted in the field are:

(1) **Plain Chlorination:** As the name suggested in this type of chlorination there is only chlorine is added to the water and no other types of treatment is required. The raw water is directly supplied to distribution pipes by adding chlorine. The source of raw water should be cleaned and do not have turbidity greater than 30 mg/l. this type of chlorination can be used in time of emergency when full-fledged water treatment is not possible. The amount of chlorine added in this method should be around 0.5 mg/l.

(2) **Pre-chlorination:** In pre-chlorination, chlorine is added to raw water before filtration and rather before sedimentation and sedimentation with coagulation. This method is adopted when there is large amount of pathogen and organic matter in water. This method also helps in better coagulation. The amount of chlorine added is to be such that it leaves residual chlorine of about 0.1 mg/l to 0.5 mg/l after filtration. The amount of chlorine ranges from 5 mg/l to 10 mg/l.

(3) **Post-chlorination:** This is the normal method of applying chlorine at the end of the treatment process. These steps are generally done before supplying domestic water. The quantity of chlorine added should be such that it leaves residual chlorine of 0.1 mg/l to 0.2 mg/l after having a contact time of about 20 minutes. This residual chlorine helps in disinfection of bacteria if any present in distribution pipelines.

(4) **Double chlorination:** In double chlorination the supply water is chlorinated two times. In this method, the pre-chlorination and post-chlorination both has to be done in a single treatment unit. Double chlorination is adopted when raw water has a large number of bacteria and water is highly turbid.

(5) **Break-point chlorination:** Break-point chlorination gives us the exact idea how much amount of chlorine is required for disinfection. Any further added chlorine will remain as residual chlorine. When chlorine is added to water two different processes occur in it. In the first step, the added chlorine kills the bacteria, and some chlorine mixes with ammonia to form chloramines. After a few minutes the residual chlorine start to increase as shown in figure 2.19 from point a to b. In the second step after the pathogenic bacteria killed the residual chlorine further added chlorine will be utilized for the oxidizing of organic matter present in the water this step is shown by point c in figure 2.19. Beyond point c any added chlorine will be residual chlorine and this point is known as break-point chlorination.

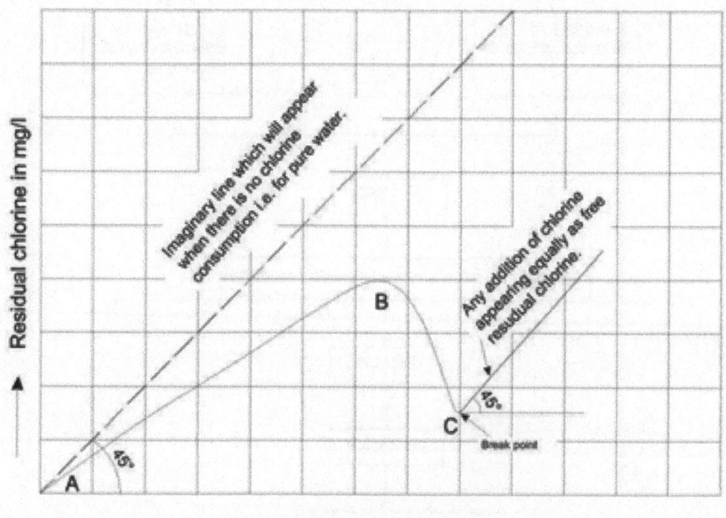

Figure 2.19: Break point chlorination

(6) **Super chlorination:** Super chlorination is to add high chlorine in water typically greater than 10 mg/l. This is to be done when there is an epidemic due to waterborne disease. In this, the residual chlorine in water after the break-point achieved in the range of 1 mg/l to 2 mg/l.

2.7.4 Residual chlorine and its importance

The amount of chlorine left in the water after all the pathogenic bacteria are killed and organic matter oxidizes is known as residual chlorine. Residual chlorine in the range of 0.1 mg/l to 0.5 mg/l should always be available in distribution pipes as it helps in protecting water from any type of infection from bacteria.

Various tests are conducted in the laboratory to find residual chlorine in water. The most important and widely used is the orthotolidine test. In this test, 100 ml of chlorinated water is taken after the required contact time, and 1 ml of orthotolodine is added in it. The water sample will give a yellow color indicated the free or combined chlorine is available. The yellow color which occurred after adding orthotolodine is compared with the standard color available in lab and compares it to known the amount. The more yellowish color indicated the more amount of residual chlorine present in water. If the distribution pipe water gives lemon color it means it is safe for drinking.

2.7.5 Flow diagram of water treatment plants

Figure 2.20 shows the flow diagram of the water treatment plant. The different process mention in flow chart is explained in the above mention text.

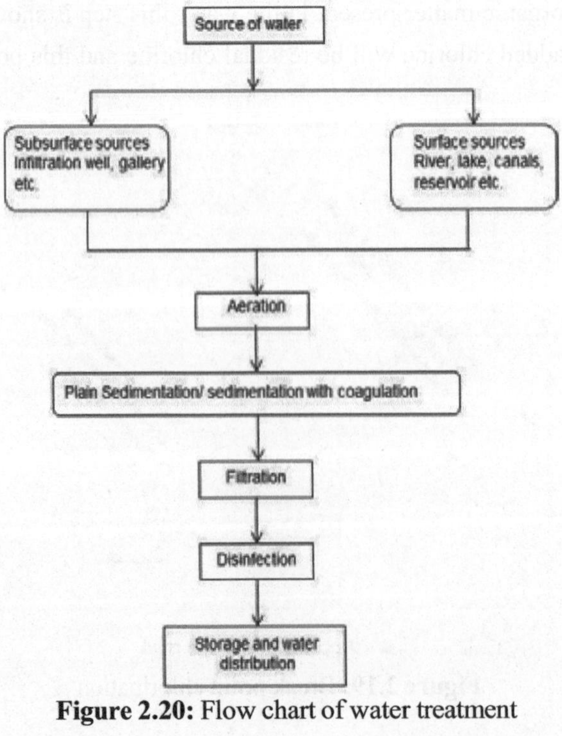

Figure 2.20: Flow chart of water treatment

2.8 Miscellaneous water treatments

The main water treatment units such as sedimentation, sedimentation with coagulation, filtration, and disinfection are described in detail in the above-mentioned section. Some other treatment units are also used for water treatment such as softening and defluoridation techniques used for removing hardness and fluoride from raw water. This method helps in correction taste and odor of water and is explained in below mention section.

2.8.1 Introduction to water softening

Softening is a process in which hardness is removed from water. Softening is not always used in the treatment process as supplying water is not much hard and it cannot cause any harm to humans. Softening helps in lowering the cost of soap consumption as well as it enhances the taste of water. When the water has to be supplied for industrial purpose then softening is very useful as hard water can cause scaling in boiler and in drying industries can cause stain on clothes.

There are two types of hardness in water one is temporary hardness due to carbonate and noncarbonated compounds of sodium and calcium while permanent hardness is due to sulphate and chloride compounds. Temporary hardness are removed by boiling of water and adding lime while permanent hardness removed by ion exchange process and zeolite process.

2.8.2 Defluoridation techniques

Defluorination means the removal of excess fluoride from raw water. If there is fluoride present above permissible limit in water it can it can adversely affect the human health by degrading the teeth and bones. Different techniques are developed over time for fluoride removal. These methods are:

(a) **Adsorption techniques:** In this techniques fluoride ions are get adsorbed on activated carbon, activated alumina and bone char. In this method the water which contain fluoride are passed through this activated particle or these activated particles are mixed with fluoride water. Fluoride ions are adsorbed on the surface of this activated particle by chemical or physical interactions. Activated particle are to be regenerated after complete removal of fluoride for again defluoridation. This method helps in removing other contaminants as well.

(b) **Ion exchange techniques:** In this method the resins are used for ion exchange the fluoride ion with these ions available in this resin. In this method the resins are choosing is such a way that it has high fondness with fluoride ions and can easily ion exchange take place. The resins are collected in a tank and water is allowed to pass through it. This method is highly effective in remove fluoride but its initial cost is very high.

(c) **Precipitation technique:** This is the most common technique used for removal of fluoride ions. This technique is also known as Nalgonda technique. This technique is developed by National Environmental Engineering Research Institute, Nagpur. In this method different chemical are added in a sequence after which flocculation is done for rapid mixing of chemical. Rapid mixing is done for

30 sec to 60 sec at 10 to 30 rpm. This flocculated water is passed in a sedimentation tank where large flocculate containing fluoride ions are settling at the bottom of the tank. This method is very simple and easy to design and operate. The chemicals used are easily available. This method also helps in removal of color, odor and taste.

UNIT SUMMARY

- Raw water which is supplied after the water treatment unit is known as purified water.
- Aeration is done to remove dissolved gases.
- Aeration helps removing iron and manganese.
- Different aeration processes are spray nozzle method, cascade method, air diffusion method and trickling bed method.
- Plain sedimentation is done to remove suspended particles heavier than water.
- Very fine suspended particle are removed with the help of coagulation
- With the help of coagulation the particle size increase and become heavier and settle at the bottom of sedimentation tank.
- Various coagulants are used for treatment are alum, ferrous sulphate, ferric sulphate, sodium aluminate.
- Jar test is done to find out the optimum coagulant dose required for the treatment plant.
- Sedimentation tank based on flows are intermittent flow and continuous flow.
- Different zones in sedimentation tanks are inlet. Outlet, sludge and settling zone.
- Clariflocculator is at type of tank in which both coagulation and flocculation take place.
- Different mechanism involve infiltration are mechanical straining, sedimentation, biological action and electrolytic changes.
- Various filter used in domestic water treatment are slow sand filter, rapid sand filter and pressure filter.
- Rapid sand filter are generally used in large town where a large volume of water is required.
- Pressure filter are like small rapid sand filter which is placed inside the closed vessel and operate under high pressure.
- Different problems occur in filtration are air binding, mud balls formation and cracking a filters.
- Disinfection helps in killing and destroying all pathogenic bacteria and also helps in maintain water free from bacteria.
- Various method of disinfection are available which helps in destabilizing bacteria.
- Chlorine is best disinfection and generally used as its leave residual chlorine.
- Chlorine can be used in powder for, gas form as well as liquid form.
- Chlorine can be added in water treatment at different stages depending on the sources of raw water.
- Softening of water is done to remove permanent as well as temporary hardness from water.

- Different defluoridation techniques used for removal of fluoride from water
- Nalgonda techniques is used major in India for removal of excess fluoride from water.

EXERCISES

Multiple Choice Questions

1. Various method of aeration?

   (a) Spray nozzle method (b) Cascade method

   (c) Trickling bed method (d) All of the above

2. In slow sand filtration, the rate of filtration should be

   (a) 100 to 200 liter/hr/m^2 (b) 100 to 150 liter/hr/m^2

   (c) 200 to 300 liter/hr/m^2 (d) 100 to 250 liter/hr/m^2

3. Which test is to done to find out the optimum dose of coagulant to treat raw water?

   (a) Turbidity test (b) Jar test

   (c) Ortholidine test (d) None

4. Which of the following does help in disinfection of water:

   (a) Alum (b) chlorine

   (c) Filtration (d) Both (a) and (b)

5. Sedimentation with coagulation is required when turbidity is more than

   (a) 30 to 40 mg/l (b) 20 to 30 mg/l

   (c) 10 to 20 mg/l (d) 15 to 25 mg/l

6. In rapid sand filtration the uniform coefficient of sand should be

   (a) 1.1 m to 1.5 m (b) 1.3 m to 1.7 m

   (c) 2.1 m to 2.7 m (d) 2.3 m to 2.7 m

7. What pressure to be kept for pressure filtration process?

   (a) 500 KN/m_2 to 800 KN/m^2 (b) 400 KN/m^2 to 600 KN/m^2

   (c) 300 KN/m_2 to 700 KN/m^2 (d) None of the above

8. What are the problems occur in filtration operation?

   (a) Mechanical Straining (b) Air binding

   (c) Biological action (d) None

9. Which test is done to measure residual chlorine in laboratory?

   (a) Jar Test (b) Orthotolidine

   (c) Both (a) and (b) (d) None

10. Different mechanism of filtration are

    (a) Mechanical Straining (b) Sedimentation

    (c) Electrolytic changes (d) All of the above

Answers of Multiple Choice Questions

1. (d), 2. (a), 3. (b), 4. (b), 5. (a), 6. (b), 7. (c), 8. (b), 9. (b) 10. (d)

Short and Long Answer Type Questions

1. Why is water aeration required? How does this method take place?
2. Write a short note on trickling bed method and cascade method.
3. Describe the principle of sedimentation tank.
4. Name the various zones of the continuous flow sedimentation tank with neat diagram and explain the working.
5. Write briefly about hopper bottom sedimentation tank.
6. Explain the various coagulant use in water treatment
7. Explain the test that is done to determine the optimal dose of coagulant.
8. Explain the difference between coagulation and flocculation
9. Describe the principle of coagulation
10. Explain the difference between slow sand filtration and rapid sand filtration
11. Explain the working and construction of pressure filter
12. What is the function of under drain pipe in filtration?
13. Why is compressed air used when washing rapid sand filter?
14. What are the operational problem occur in filtration?
15. Write short note on under drain of rapid sand filtration.
16. Explain the various method of disinfection.
17. Write a short note on break point chlorination and super chlorination.
18. What is meant by softening of water?
19. Highlight the need of defluoridation. Explain various techniques used.
20. Explain different between pre chlorination and post chlorination.

REFERENCES AND SUGGESTED READINGS

1. Garg, S.K., Environmental Engineering Vol. I and Vol. II, Khanna Publishers
2. Sharma S.C, Environmental Engineering, Khanna Publishing House, New Delhi
3. Punmia, B C, Environmental Engineering, vol. I and II, Laxmi Publishers
4. Basak N N, Environmental Engineering, McGraw Hill Publishers.

3 Conveyance and Distribution of Water

UNIT SPECIFICS

Through this unit we have discussed the following aspects:

- *To understand and select suitable pipe material for water supply*
- *DIfferent types of water joints and valves*
- *Different method for distribution of water*
- *Overview of services reservoir*
- *To understand the layouts of distribution of water pipes for water supply*

To help the students in the visualization of the content and to enhance their practical knowledge, the figures are provided in 2D. The content in this unit offers practical knowledge and will help the students in decision-making during the fieldwork.

This unit contains short and long answer-type questions along with multiple choice questions, a list of references, and suggested reading so that one can go through them for practice. Some QR codes are given which can be scanned for more information on various topics of interest and to get extra knowledge.

RATIONALE

This unit on the conveyance and distribution of water helps the students to develop an idea about the various types of pipes used for conveyance of water. It explains to select suitable pipe material for a particular type of water supply. The various pipe materials used for the water supply are discussed. A brief discussion of various types of water joints is explained. The various water valves are also discussed and their uses and location are well explained. The different method of distribution of water is discussed. The content covered in this unit is important to understand the conveyance and distribution of water for water supply schemes.

The knowledge of various conveyance and distribution systems of water is essential for civil engineering students. The students can apply the knowledge of the designing water distribution mains and branches for water supply. The knowledge gained in this unit will help the students to identify suitable types of joints and valves to be used at particular condition in water supply scheme. The students can apply their knowledge in the selection and implementation of desired layout of distribution system. The concepts in this unit will help the student in effective supervision of laying a suitable water distribution lines for water supply.

PRE-REQUISITES

A basic knowledge of different material and sources of water is required.

UNIT OUTCOMES

The list of outcomes of this unit is as follows:

U3-O1: *To learn how to select suitable pipe material.*

U3-O2: *To understand the various water pipe joints and valves.*

U3-O3: *To learn method of distribution of water.*

U3-O4: *To determine layout of distribution of water.*

U3-O5: *To propose suitable service reservoirs.*

Unit-3 Outcomes	EXPECTED MAPPING WITH COURSE OUTCOMES (1- Weak Correlation; 2- Medium correlation; 3- Strong Correlation)				
	CO-1	CO-2	CO-3	CO-4	CO-5
U3-O1	1	-	2	-	-
U3-O2	1	1	2	-	-
U3-O3	1	1	3	-	-
U3-O4	1	-	3	-	-
U3-O5	1	-	3	-	-

3.1 Conveyance

In the previous unit, you got the idea about different water treatment units and their principle and mechanism on which these treatment units work. After the water is got treated it has to be transferred from the treatment unit to the storage tank and from there to the distribution system for supply to the individual households. In the conveyance system the water is transported in two stages the first one is from sources to the treatment unit and the other stage is from the treatment unit to industrial, domestic, and commercial purposes. The water is transported under gravity or by pressure depends on the location and elevation of the sources and treatment unit in first stage and in latter stage it depends on the location and elevation of the town or city from treatment units.

Conveyance depending on the flow of pipe is of two types. They are:

(1) Gravity Conveyance: In gravity conveyance water flows under the influence of gravitational force. In this the water source is having higher elevation as compared to place where water has to be supplied. In this type of water supply pipeline, the hydraulic gradient line is at same level with the water surface and this hydraulic gradient line remains parallel to the bottom surface of the conveyance as shown in figure 3.1. In gravity conduct the water remains under atmospheric pressure and in Bernoulli's theorem there is no such pressure exist.

The bottom of such conveyance always follows the hydraulic gradient line which helps in controlling the flow velocity. In this type of conveyance natural available slope cannot be followed as the conduit cannot be laid upside down and in valleys according to the natural topography of the area. Gravity conveyance can be made in the form of a canal channel or aqueduct.

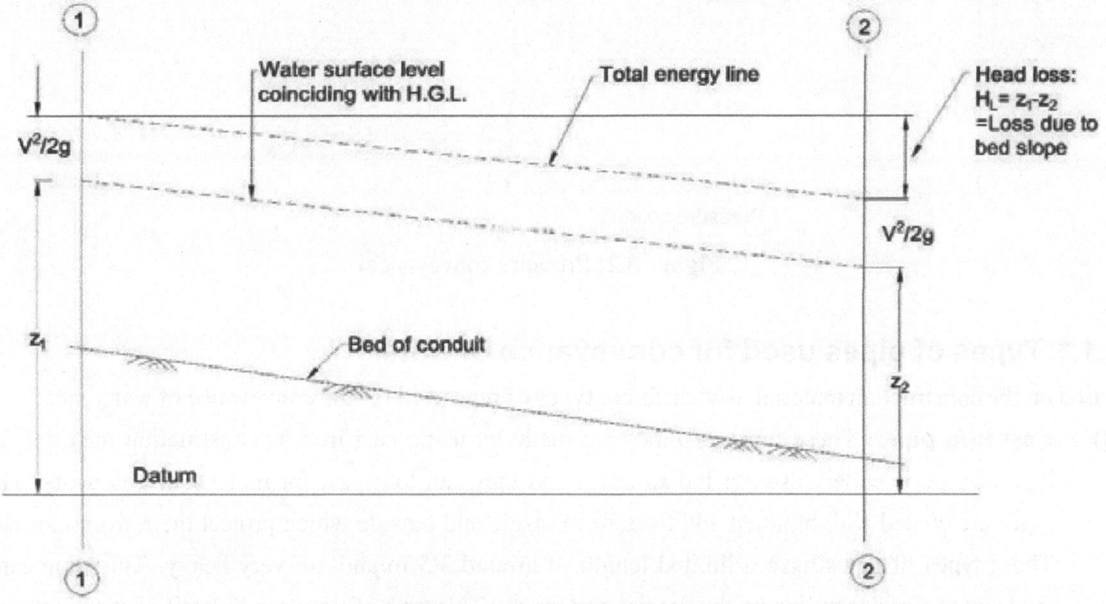

Figure 3.1: Gravity conveyance

(2) **Pressure Conveyance:** Pressure conveyance is a closed pipe in which water flow under pressure and no air is allowed to come inside. In this type of conveyance, the pressure is above atmospheric pressure. In this type of conveyance, the hydraulic gradient line is formed by calculating the desired elevation at different points using piezometer tubes as shown in figure 3.2. In pressure conduct, the bottom slope is independent of the hydraulic gradient line. These types of conduct are free to follow natural gradients and can easily pass through mountains and valleys.

Pressure conveyance is much easier to construct as compare to gravity conveyance and are economical as they can follow the shorter path to reach the water to their desired location. There is another advantage of using pressure conduct is that they are not exposed to atmosphere so there is no chance of getting contaminated while water is transport from one place to another. Pressure conveyance is globally used to transport water.

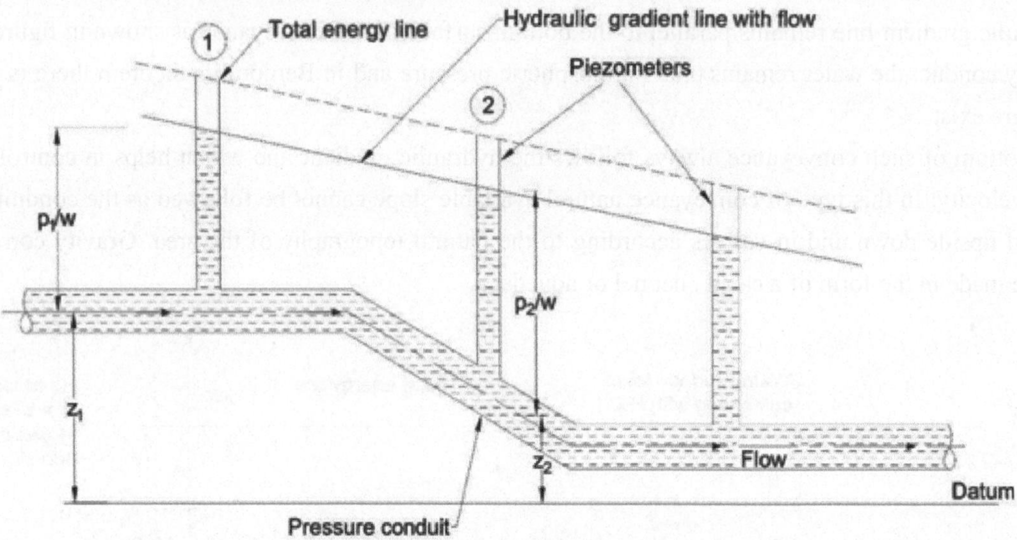

Figure 3.2: Pressure conveyance

3.1.1 Types of pipes used for conveyance of water

Based on the construction material used different types of pipe used for the conveyance of water are:

(a) **Cast iron pipes:** These types of pipes are made by using cast iron as construction material. This type of pipe is widely used in Indian cities and they can long last for more than 100 years. These pipes are coated with bitumen additives from inside and outside which protect them from corrosion. These types of pipes have a limited length of around 3.5 m and are very heavy. This pipe can be made up to 6 m depending on the special conditions. This type of pipe can be easily cut and joined by using socket and spigot joints. Cast iron pipes are laid underground by digging a trench or directly on the ground and are used for main water supply pipelines and major branches.

Two different methods are there for manufacturing cast iron pipes. One is sand moulding and the other one is centrifugal casting. The later centrifugal casting is lighter and more durable than the sand moulding type. In India, as per IS code 1536-1976 centrifugal casting pipes are classified into three types based on working pressure. They are Class 1A (working pressure 1200 KN/m^2), Class A (working pressure 1800 KN/m^2) and Class B (working pressure 2000 KN/m^2).

(b) **Steel Pipe:** These pipes are manufactured using steel plates of various thicknesses depending on the pressure it has to withstand are rolled to various diameters and their edges are joint by welding or riveted. Generally, welding is preferred over riveted joints as welding provides smoother and stronger joints. Steel pipes are lightweight and can withstand high pressure but can easily get corroded. These pipes are coated with bitumen additives from the inside as well as outside to protect them from acid or bases.

Steel pipes are used for the main water supply, inverted siphon, and in the place where high pressure is to be exerted on water pipes. These pipes cannot be used in distribution networks as they are difficult to join. Steel pipes can be produce up to 5m and so on their length depends on the length of the rolling steel plate which kept up to 11 m in length.

(c) **Galvanized Iron Pipes:** These pipes are made up of wrought iron coated with zinc to protect it from corrosion. In this pipe, thread can be easily made and can be easily joined. This pipe has an age of around 15 years. This pipe is joined by using a screwed and socked joint arrangement. These pipes are made up of smaller diameter and are used in household fitting and distribution network. These pipes are also known as service pipes as they are used in- house. These pipe diameters vary from 13 mm to 100 mm and have lengths of around 7 m.

(d) **Cement Concrete pipe:** These pipes are made up of plain cement concrete of size up to 60 cm in diameter. These pipe can be made on site using cement, concrete and sand known as cast-in situ and can be transport from other manufacturing site known as pre-cast. Concrete cement pipes are very heavy and they are difficult to transport. These pipes are not used to transport high-pressure water.

(e) **Reinforced Cement Concrete pipe:** Reinforced cement concrete pipes are produced using thin steel wires or steel bars inserted inside the cement concrete pipe which increases the strength of the pipe. Reinforced cement concrete pipe can be made up to 2 m in diameter. Reinforced cement concrete pipe can be manufactured by pouring the cement contrite mixture in the mould having steel bars, after complete pouring curing is to be done to attain proper strength. In another method, cement concrete mixture is poured in mould containing steel bars that are rotated so that uniform layers of cement concrete lay over the bars. The quantity of steel bars is around 0.25 % of the circumference area of the pipe. The reinforced cement concrete pipe are made using the provision given in IS code 458-2021. These pipes are used in the main distribution supply. These pipes can take compressive load and do not collapse on normal traffic load. These pipes have a life span of around 75 years and are cheap.

(f) **Hume Steel Pipe:** Hume steel pipes are type of steel pipes which is coated with cement mortar from inside and outside. The thicknesses of cement coating depend on the diameter of the pipe which generally varies from 1.25 cm to 3.80 cm. The diameter of this pipe varies from 10 cm to 180 cm having a length of around 2.5 m. This pipe is heavy and difficult to transport. They are used in the distribution of water in the water supply scheme.

(g) **Asbestos cement pipe:** These pipes are made up material such as silica, cement and asbestos which are compressed under pressure to make a homogenous mixture of asbestos which have high strength. This pipe is light in weight and fire resistance. They are rust-free. These pipes are available in different diameter ranges from 5 cm to 90 cm and have a length of approximately 4 m. They can handle the pressure up to 25 Kg/cm^2. Socket and spigot joint arrangement is used to join the smaller diameter asbestos pipe while large diameter pipe is join using collar joint method. This pipe is not much used in water supply scheme as it contains harmful asbestos material.

(h) **Plastic pipes:** These pipes are now very common to use for water supply at home. This pipe is light in weight, durable, and rust-free. They are easy to transport and can be easily cut and joined. This pipe cannot handle temperatures above 60°C. These pipes can be made of different diameter which varies from 2 cm to 30 cm and have a length of 6 m. They can withstand pressure up to 10 kg/cm^2. Different types of plastic pipe such as low-density polyethylene, high- density polyethylene and un-plasticized are available in the market and are made using provisions laid in IS 3076:1985(R2003), IS 4984:1995(R2002) and IS 4985:2000 respectively.

3.1.2 Choice of Pipe Material

The choice of pipe material for the water supply scheme depends on the following points:

- Flowing water properties and its quantity
- The amount of water pipe can carry and transport
- Material strength and pipe durability
- Life span of the pipe
- Pipe material cost
- Easy to transport the pipe
- Pipe fitting and other materials available in the market
- Expenses of repair work of pipe and protection
- Difficult in laying pipe

For higher pressure water and larger diameter the steel pipes are used to transport water. When the water pressure is normal cast iron and reinforced cement concrete pipe is used. For branches and distribution, the cast iron pipe is preferred. In domestic and household water supply galvanized iron pipe and plastic pipe is used.

3.1.3 Types of Joints

Pipes are available in smaller lengths generally 2 m to 6 m. To increase their length the pipe are connected to get the desired length. Different types of joints which are used to get the desired length are given below:

(1) Socket and Spigot Joint: Cast iron pipes are joined by these types of joints along the length as they form permanent joints. In this type of joint one end of the joint is larger than the pipe diameter the other side is the same as the diameter of the pipe. The larger side opening is known as a socket while the other side opening is known as a spigot. The spigot end is wrapped with jute cloth before inserting in the socket side. The space left between the spigot and socket is filled with molten leads which on cooling become solidified and make the waterproof joint. Around 3.5 kg lead is required for 150 mm diameter pipe for making water tight and leak proof joint. These types of joints are flexible and can be laid on the ground which is curved and somewhat flat. To install this type of joint there is a requirement of skilled labor. Figure 3.3 shows the socket and spigot joint.

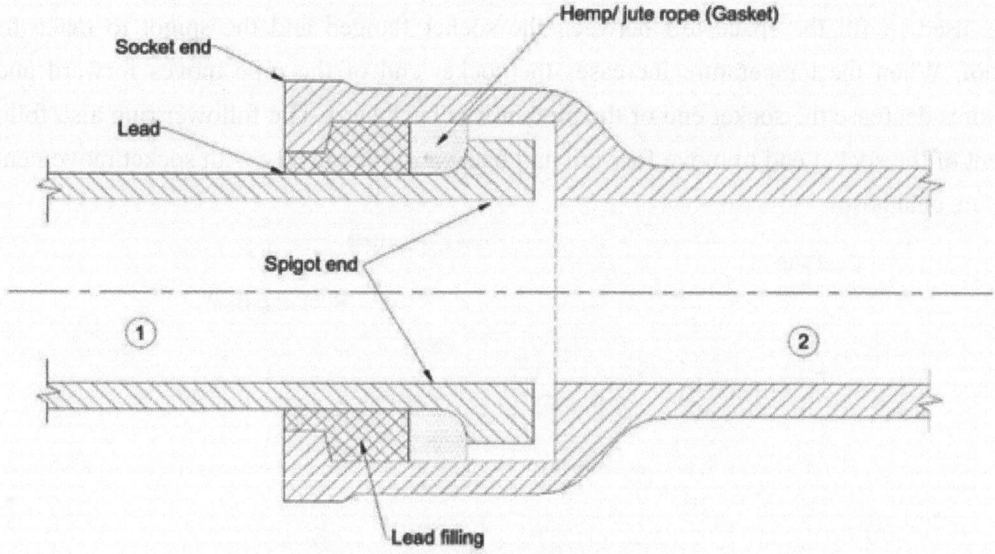

Figure 3.3: Socket and spigot joint

(2) Flanged joint: This type of joint is used in water treatment plant where there is pipe are to be disjoint latter after joining. This joint is strong and durable. Flanged joints are very useful in places where there is temperature occur. Flanged joints are mostly used in steel pipes. In a flanged joint the flange is made at the both end and this flanged is joint by using bolts which installed in the flanges. Rubber or gasket is kept between the flange to make them water proof as shown in figure 3.4. These types of joints are expensive and generally used for indoor work.

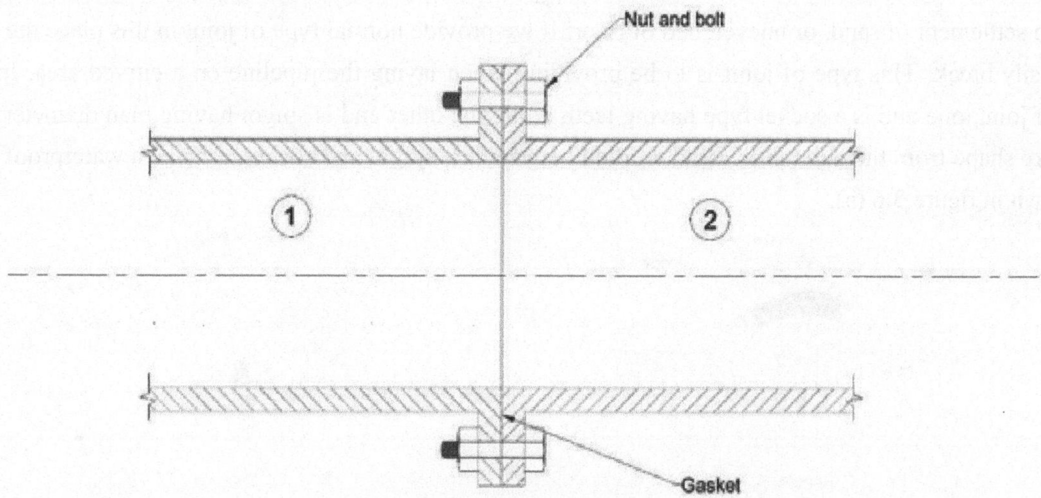

Figure 3.4: Flanged joint

(3) Expansion joint: Expansion joints are given in pipelines which are changed in length due to thermal expansion caused by atmospheric temperature variation. Expansion joints are mainly used in cast iron pipes in which socket ends are flanged while the other end of the pipe is normally spigot. Nuts and bolts are used to tighten the socket flanged with a cast iron follower ring as shown in figure 3.5. The rubber gasket is used to fill the space left between the socket flanged and the spigot to make the joint waterproof. When the temperature increases the socket end of the pipe moves forward and when temperatures decrease the socket end of the pipe moves backward. The follower ring also follows the movement of the socket end to move forward and backward receptively with socket movement as the temperature changes.

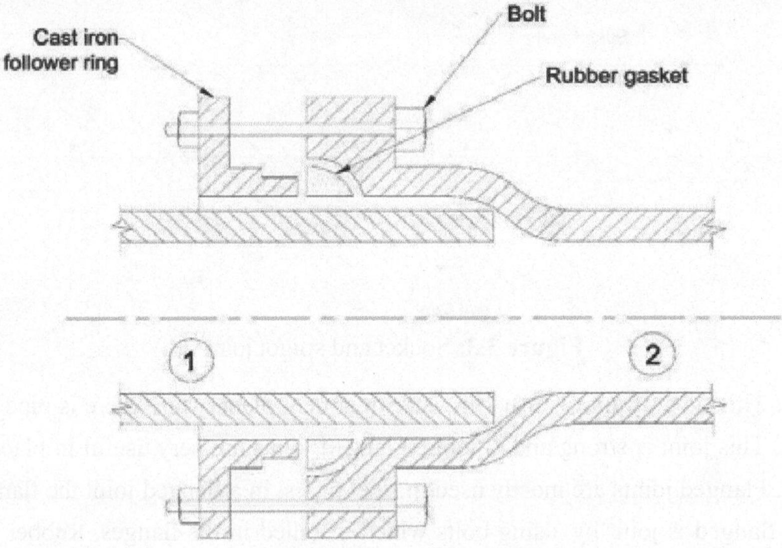

Figure 3.5: Expansion joint

(4) Flexible joint: Flexible joint is provided in the pipes where there is flexibility required due to soft land, uneven settlement of sand, or uneven bed of river. If we provide normal type of joint in this place the joint can easily break. This type of joint is to be providing when laying the pipeline on a curved area. In this type of joint, one end is a socket type having teeth while the other end is spigot having plan diameter with bell-like shape from the outer side. Lead is filled between the spigot and socket to make a waterproof joint as shown in figure 3.6 (a).

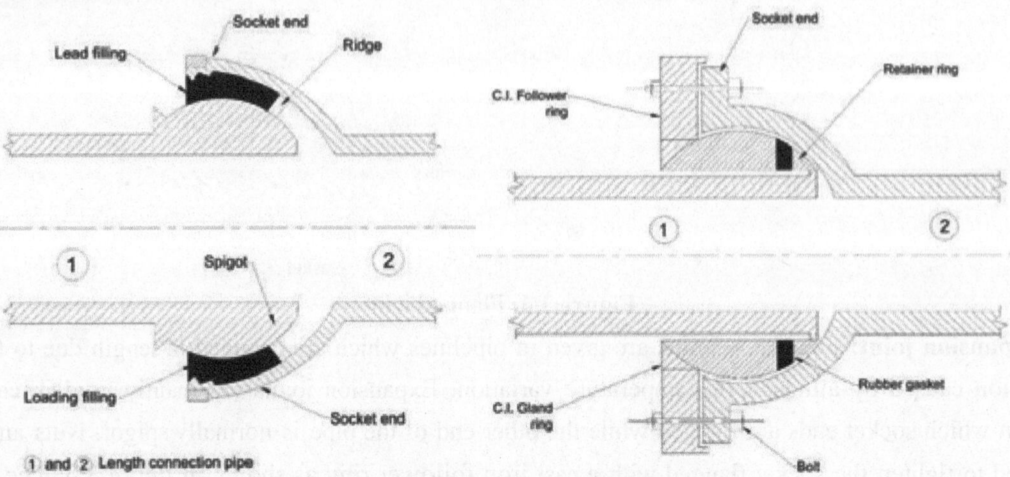

Figure 3.6: (a) and (b) Flexible joint

There is another type of flexible joint in which the spigot is circular in shape and a retainer ring is placed between the socket and the spigot. The cast iron gland ring is attached to the socket end with the help of a nut and bolt as shown in figure 3.6 (b).

(5) Coupling joint: Coupling joint is used to join cast iron pipe when it pipe has to move over the bridge or it has to pass below the bridge. This joint is strong and water-resistant. They are rigid and do not break due to vibration in the pipe. In this joint both the pipes have a plain diameter and a special type of middle ring is attached between the follower ring as shown in figure 3.7. The gasket is provided between the pipe and middle ring to make water proof joint. The follower ring is connected with the help of nuts and bolts.

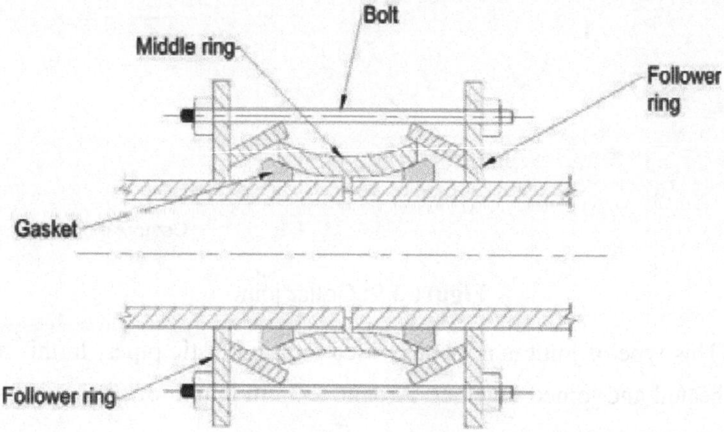

Figure 3.7: Coupling joint

(6) Screwed and socket joint: This type of joint is used to connect galvanized iron pipe and steel pipe of small diameter. This joint is used to connect distribution pipes in-house as it is easy to cut thread on this pipe. In this joint the thread is cut on the outer surface of the pipe and they are joined by thread socket as shown in figure 3.8. A cotton thread is rubbed on the surface of the pipe before the joint to make it water leak-proof. This type of joint can be easy to remove and install. There is difficult to joint large diameter pipe by this method as it is not possible to make thread on their end.

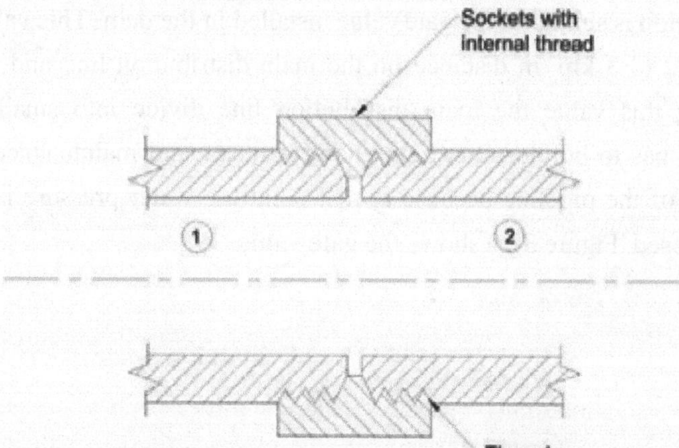

Figure 3.8: Screwed and socket joint

(7) Collar joint: Collar joints are used to join Hume pipes of larger diameter. In the collar joint, both pipes have the same diameter. In this joint pipe end are placed face to face and a gasket is placed between the two ends. A collar is placed above both ends of the pipe and cement mortar is filled between the collar and pipe as shown in figure 3.9.

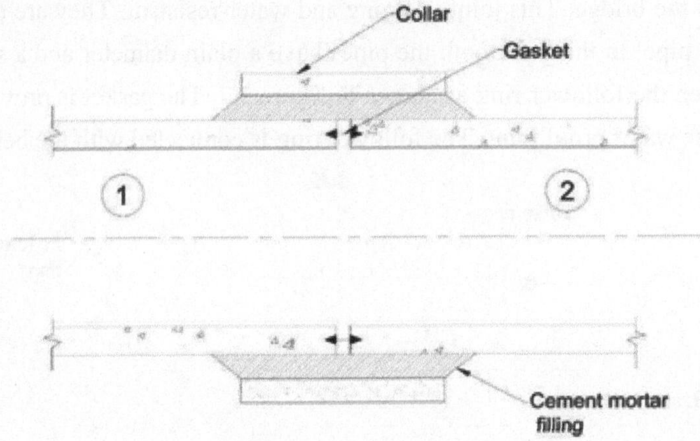

Figure 3.9: Collar joint

(8) Welding Joint: This type of joint is now days used to join plastic pipes. In this method, both ends of the plastic pipe are heated and joined together. Around 2-3 cm length of pipe is heated and covered with solvent is clamped into another pipe.

3.1.4 Types of Valves

Valves are provided in the pipeline to control the velocity of flow of water and to repair and cleaning of the pipeline. They also help in changing the direction of the flow of water. These values are provided at suitable intervals and particular points according to their use and function in a pipeline. Different types of valves are there as per their use and function. They are explained in the below-mentioned paragraph.

(a) Gate valve: This type of value helps in the regulation of the flow of water by controlling the flow in the pipeline. Their function is similar to the gate value installed in the dam. This value is generally installed at an interval of about 2 to 3 km in distance on the main distribution line and at the cross junction of branches. By installing this value the main distribution line divide into small section and only that particular section value has to be closed at both ends for repair and maintenance work. Gate valves are installed at the summit of the pipeline because at that point the water pressure is low and the value can easily be opened and closed. Figure 3.10 shows the gate value.

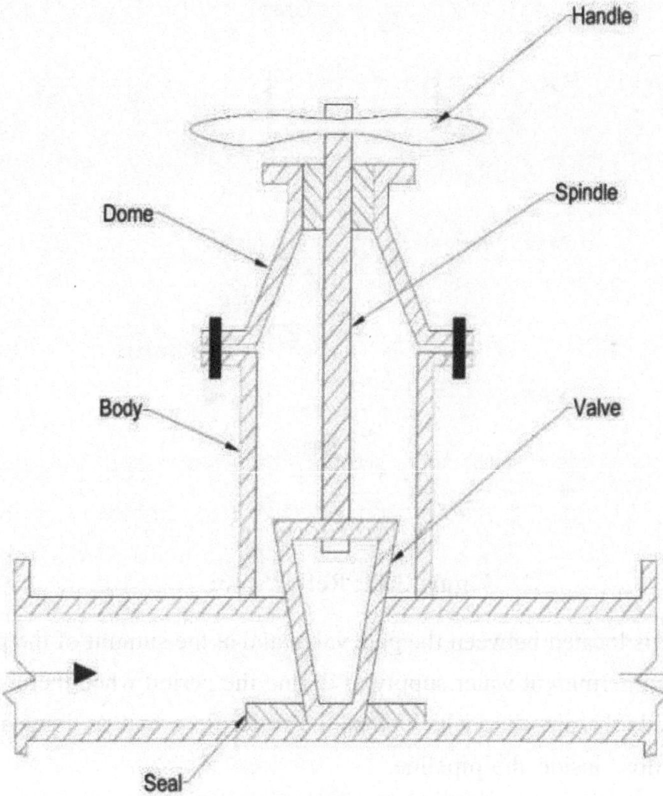

Figure 3.10: Gate valve

The outer part is made using cast iron and the inner part is made using brass and steel material. In the gate valve, the inside valve is attached to the spindle which is ultimately attached to the handle as shown in figure 3.10. This handle is rotated by hand manually or mechanically to move the valve up and down to control the flow of water. The valve is joined to the pipeline using different joint methods such as socket and spigot joint, flanged joint, and thread socket joint. There is an arrow inscribed on the pipeline to know the flow of water and easy to operate. This value has to be opened and closed once in 3 month to control the jamming of valve. This valve is also known as a sluice valve.

(b) Reflux valve or check valve: This valve is also known as a non-return valve as it allows flow of water in only one direction in the pipeline. This valve helps in controlling the backward flow of water when the pump accidentally stop working by automatically close it valve as shown in figure 3.11. This valve is installed at the foot of the overhead water tank to prevent backflow of water. The reflux value contains a flat disc which is attached to the hinge of the pipe in such a way that a one-directional flow of water is possible as shown in figure 3.11. When the flow of water is in the opposite direction this flat disc closes due to its own weight and does not open.

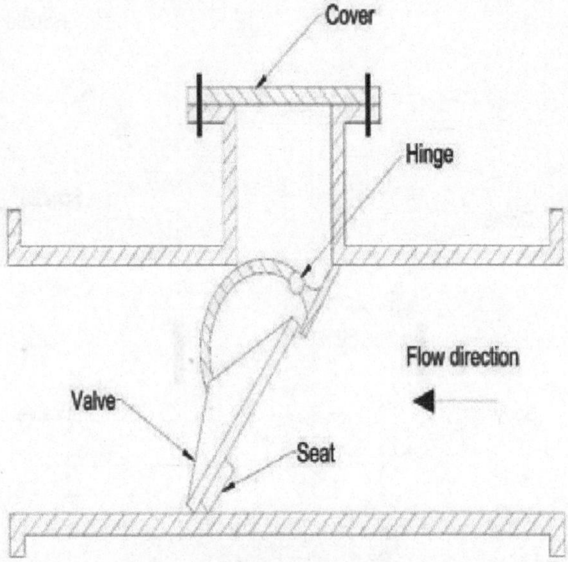

Figure 3.11: Reflux valve

(c) Air valve: This valve is located between the gate valve and at the summit of the pipeline. This value is very useful when there is intermittent water supply as during the period when there is no water flowing in the pipe the air filled inside the pipe line which stops the water flow and as long as this air is there in pipe the water will not flow inside the pipeline.

Therefore to release this filled air from the pipeline the air valve is provided in the pipeline. This value also helps in controlling the possibility of a vacuum forming inside the pipeline and helps the pipeline from bursting. This valve contains a chamber made up of cast iron, a knob, an air vent, and a floating valve as shown in figure 3.12. The cast iron chamber rectangular/circular is attached to the pipeline. When there is water in the pipeline the knob lever is struck to the air vent and make air vent is closed. As soon as the water is closed in the pipeline the water level drop in the cast iron chamber which allows the float valve to hang down and open the air vent which is closed by the knob to release any air present in the pipeline. As soon as the water flow starts the floating valve rises and the knob attached to the lever of the floating valve also rises and gets stuck to the air vent and closes the air vent. This way only air exits from the pipe and water does not escape from the pipeline. The air valve works automatically.

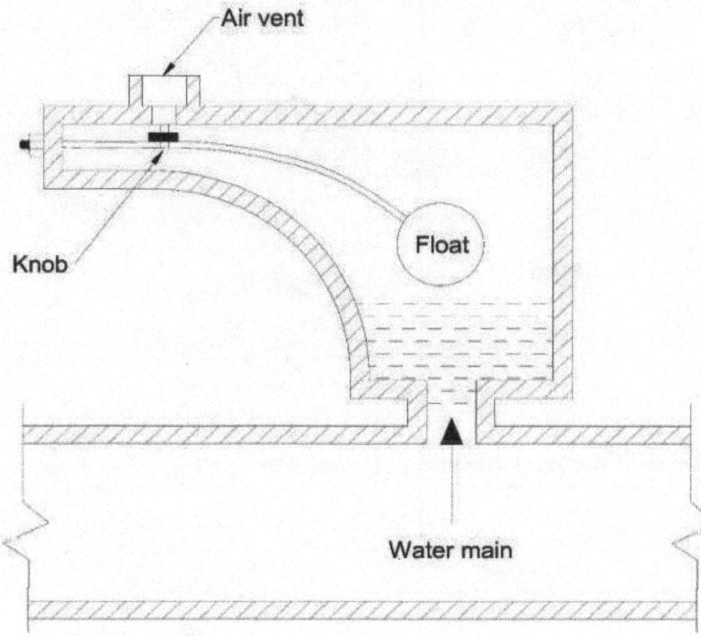

Figure 3.12: Air valve

(d) Pressure relief valve: As the name suggest this valve is useful in reducing the extra pressure from the pipeline and helps in protecting from bursting the pipe. This valve automatically opens when the water pressure inside the pipeline exceeds certain predefined pressure and releases this extra pressure by releasing the water from the pipeline it automatically closes when the extra pressure reduces to the predefined pressure. This valve is provided upstream of the gate valve because as the sluice valve suddenly closed the water hammer phenomenon will developed on the upstream and this valve helps in releasing the pressure from pipeline. This valve is made of a cast iron chamber having a spring, stem, disc, and handle as shown in figure 3.13.

In the pressure relief valve the disc is attached to the spring in such a way that at predefined pressure the disc is laid on the surface of the pipe and as the water pressure increase in the pipeline this disc moves upward direction and open the valve to release the extra water. When the pressure again drop to the predefined level the disc come download and laid on the surface of pipeline and closed the valve. This all process occurs automatically.

This valve is also known as safety valve.

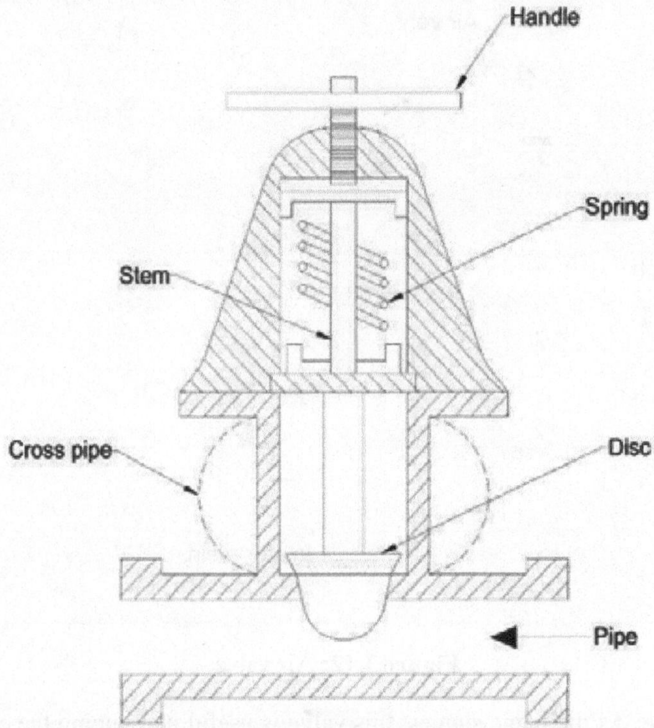

Figure 3.13: Pressure valve

(e) Scour valve: This valve is type of gate valve but they installed at the downward point of the pipeline. This valve is generally located at the branches end and ends of distribution system pipe lines. This valve helps in removing the impurities such as sand and silt from the pipeline. These impurities generally get collected at the bottom depression of the pipeline and can be removed by opening the valve at certain time intervals. This valve is also known as a drain valve and blow-off valve. This valve also helps in draining water from pipe line in case there is necessary of some repair of pipeline.

3.2 Distribution of water

After the raw water treatment, under various process, water became safe for domestic and industrial activities it now has to be transported to individual households and commercial and industrial hubs. This treated water is passed through various roads and railways to reach household of an individual. So, the function of a planned distribution system is to reach the water to each and every household and commercial and industrial hub. The distribution of the water system consists of a pipeline of different sizes, various types of valves to control the flow, and a services reservoir to store water from the treatment unit from where water is discharged into the distribution system. Distribution system must be capable to supply water continuously for 24 hour of the day and it should free from inclusion of any type of pollution. Its design should be such that it is economical and easy to repair and maintain.

3.2.1 Method of distribution of water

Different method is developed to transfer adequate water to the individual households. This method depends on the topography of the area, water source level, and water treatment plant location. The following three methods of distribution of water are based on the above conditions they are:

(1) Gravity System

(2) Pumping System

(3) Combined System

3.2.1.1 Gravity System

In this type of water distribution system, the water source such as a lake and reservoir is located at a higher point as compared to the distribution area and water merely flow under the action of gravitational force without using a pump. For the success of this type of system, there should be a proper head difference between the water source and the point where water is to be supplied so that the water available to the customer should have adequate water pressure. This type of system is very economical and reliable as there is no need for pumping at any stage of water supply. The gravity system is very successful in hilly areas where the village is located at the foothills and the water source is located top of the hills. Figure 3.14 shows the gravity system with hydraulic gradient line for static head, maximum water demand and minimum water demand.

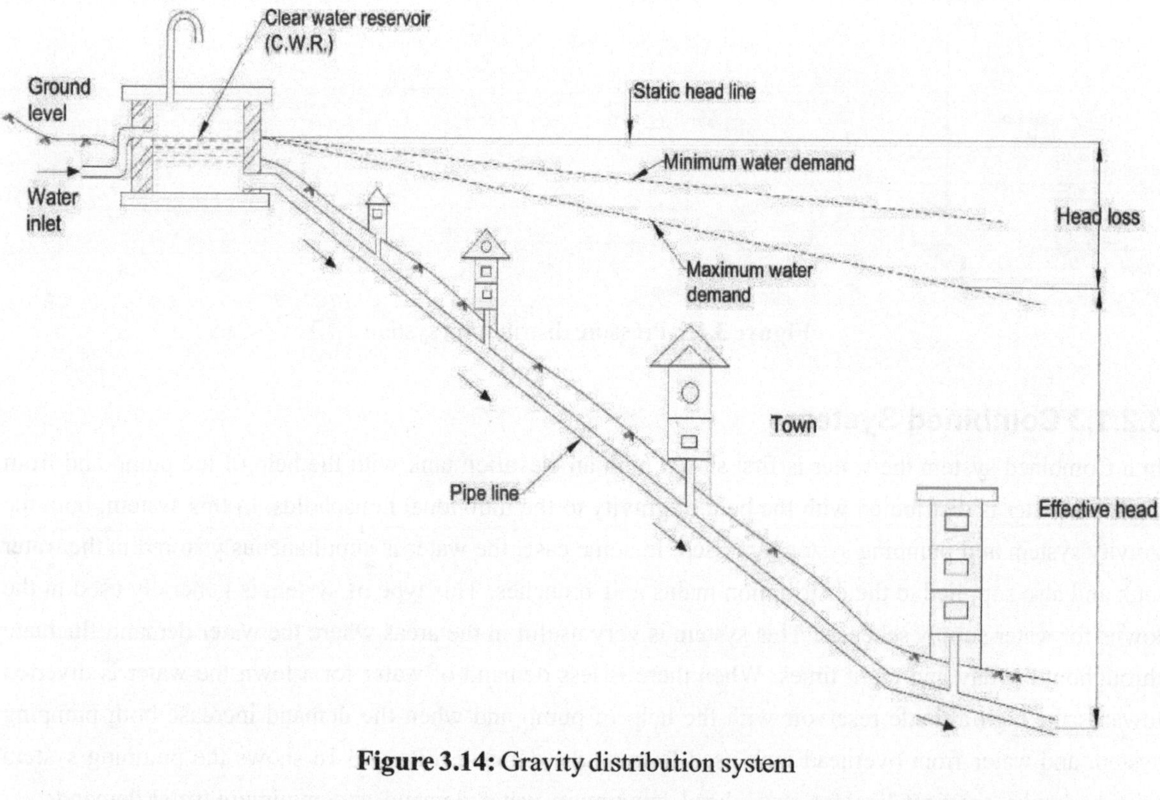

Figure 3.14: Gravity distribution system

3.2.1.2 Pumping System

In this type of water distribution system, the water treatment plant and the area to which water is to be supplied are located at same height or sometime at height above treatment unit, so it become impossible to supply water by gravity action. Then pump has to be used to provide an adequate water head to reach the desired height. In this system, there is no water storage tank is used and water is supplied directly to the consumer from the water treatment plant so this method is also known as a pumping system without storage. This pump has to be constantly monitored as there is no storage to store water. If there is so problem occurred in pump the water supply will stop in this system. The pump used in this system has to be operating at a variable head so to meet the variable demand of the household. Due to the fluctuating demand of the town extra pumping is required when demand increases. This system is expensive as pumping of water is required constantly to supply water. Figure 3.15 shows the pumping system with hydraulic gradient line for static head, maximum water demand and minimum water demand.

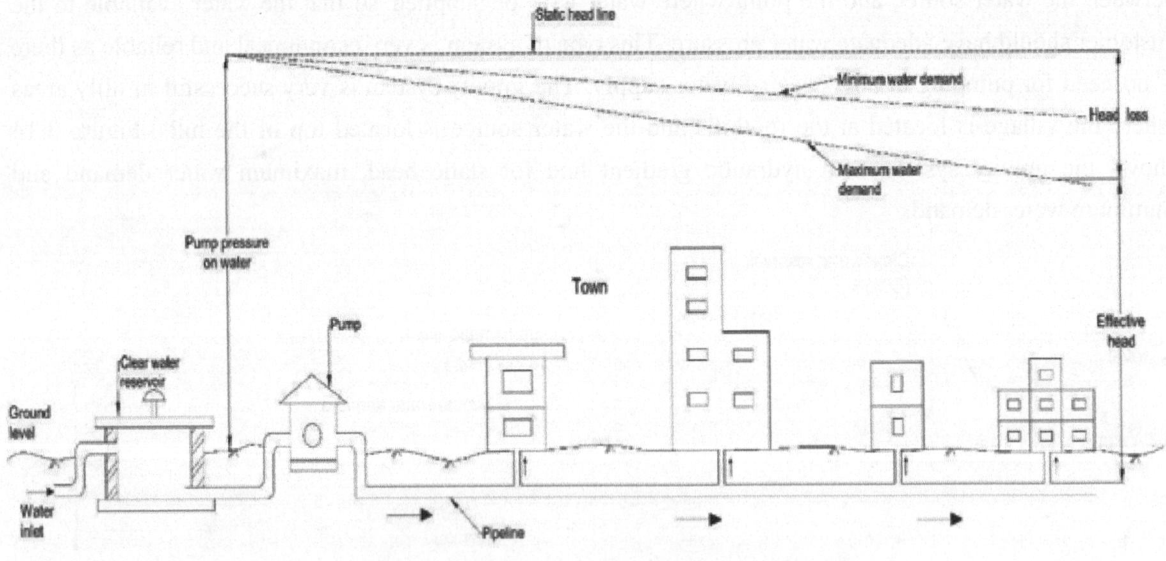

Figure 3.15: Pressure distribution system

3.2.1.3 Combined System

In a Combined system the water is first stored high an elevation tank with the help of the pump and from there the water is distributed with the help of gravity to the individual households. In this system, both the gravity system and pumping system are used. In some case, the water is simultaneously stored in the water tank and also supplied to the distribution mains and branches. This type of system is generally used in the towns for water supply schemes. This system is very useful in the areas where the water demand fluctuate throughout the day and night times. When there is less demand of water for a town the water is diverted towards the high altitude reservoir with the help of pump and when the demand increase both pumping system and water from overhead tank used to meet the demand. Figure 3.16 shows the pumping system with hydraulic gradient line for static head, maximum water demand and minimum water demand.

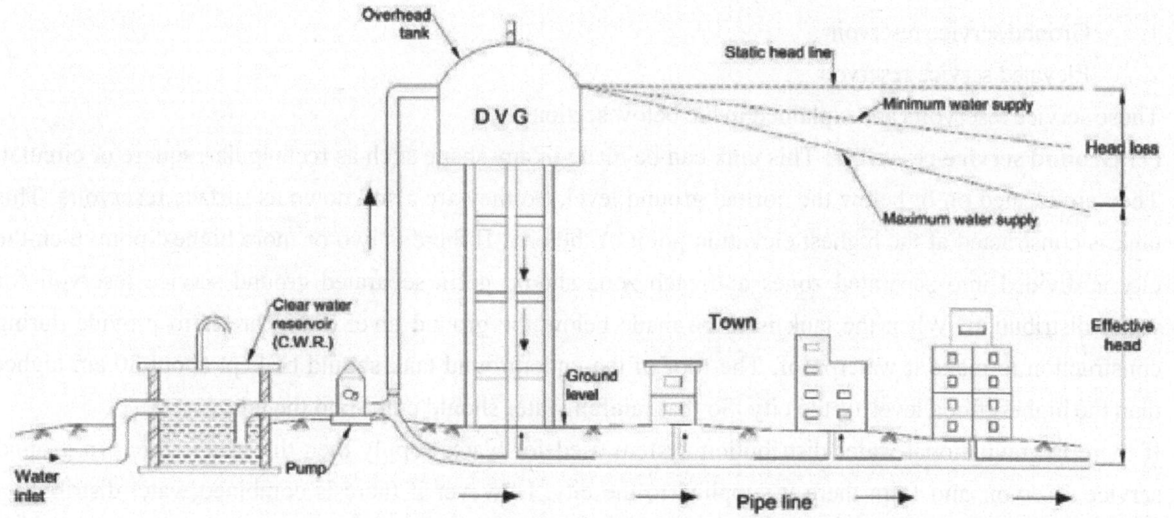

Figure 3.16: Combined distribution system

3.2.2 Service Reservoir

Service reservoirs are storage tanks that collect treated water from water treatment plants which can be used to meet the demand arising due to emergencies such as if there is any fire breakout in town or water supply is interrupted due to repairs or maintenance in water treatment plants. Service reservoirs also help to meet the fluctuation in demand occur during normal water supply. Different functions of the service reservoir are described below.

3.2.2.1 Function of service reservoir

Various utilities of a service reservoir are such as:

- This tank helps in control the fluctuation of hourly demand and maintains the water flow from water treatment plants and pumps to operate at constant flow rate which help in increase in efficiency.
- This tank helps in maintaining the constant water pressure in the distribution pipeline.
- With the help of this tank pumping can be carried out in shifts without distributing the water supply in place of running them the whole day.
- Water collected in this tank can be used in case there is any breakout of a fire incident in town.
- This tank helps decrease the operation and maintenance cost of the pump and reduces the size of pipelines.
- These tanks can be used in case a sudden defect occurs in the pump.

3.2.2.2 Types of service reservoir

The service reservoir is made up of reinforced cement concrete, cast iron, or masonry. Service reservoirs based on the location of the tank regarding the ground are classified into two types. They are:

1. Ground service reservoir
2. Elevated service reservoir

These service reservoirs are explained in the below section.

(1) Ground service reservoir: This tank can be made in any shape such as rectangular, square or circular. They are located on or below the normal ground level. So they are also known as surface reservoirs. This tank is constructed at the highest elevation point of the city. If there is two or more highest point then the city is divided into separated zones and each zone should get a separated ground service reservoir for water distribution. When the tank is to be made below the ground level extra care is to provide during construction to make it waterproof. The roof of the underground tank should be kept about 30 cm higher than the highest flood level of the city. So that rainfall water should enter into the tank.

If there is gravitational water distribution system used for water supply then the water stored in ground service reservoir and from there it supplied to the city. However if there is combined water distribution system then water is first sent to the higher elevated tank from ground service reservoir and from higher elevated tank the water distributed to the city.

Ground service reservoirs should have a flat or domed slab roof which is waterproof and should have a slope so that rainwater does not hold on the slab. The length of the ground service reservoir is kept around 1.5 times the width of the tank. The depth of the tank is kept around 2.5 m to 6 m. Ground service reservoirs have two compartments as shown in figure 3.17. In these two compartments, if one is cleaned or repaired then other tank is used for storage and water distribution. Both tanks are interconnected using gate valve at the bottom of the divided wall.

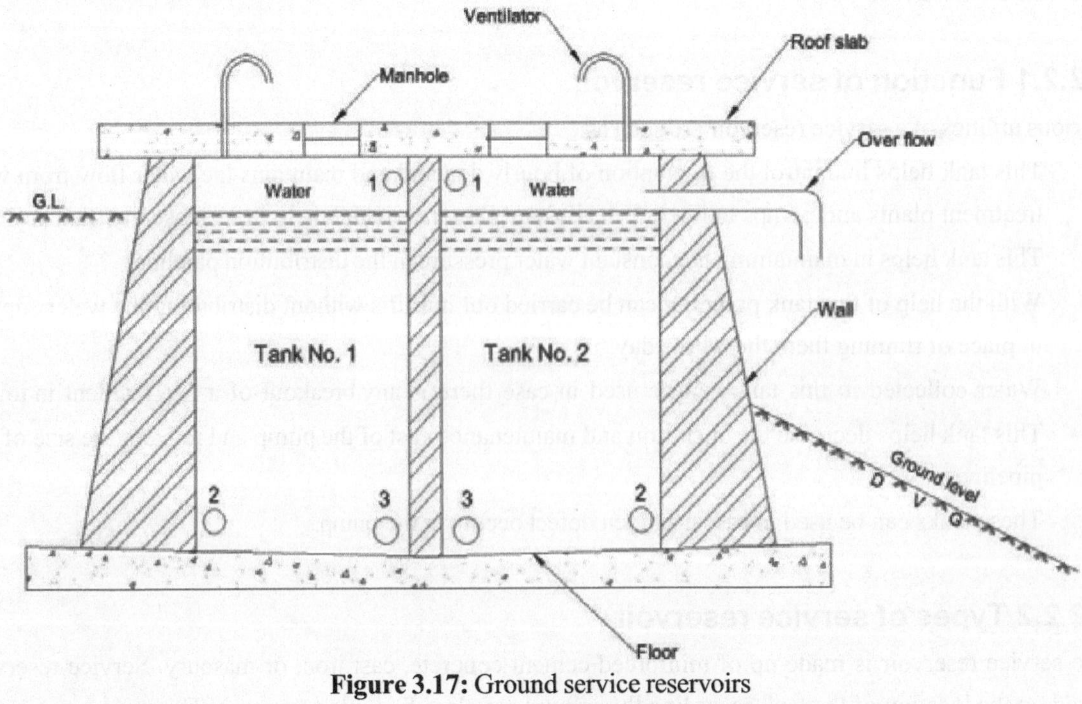

Figure 3.17: Ground service reservoirs

Each tank has an inlet pipe, outlet pipe, and washout pipe with gate valve installed on each pipe for controlling the water flow rate. Ventilation pipes are installed on the roof slab to remove contaminated air from the tank compartment. Manholes are made on the top of the tank for inspection and ladders are placed there for cleaning. Sludge from the tank is taken out from time to time from washout pipe.

(2) Elevated service reservoir: Elevated service reservoirs are made up of reinforced concrete or steel in the shape of a rectangular, circular, or intze type overhead tank which are made above the ground level with the support of staging. This tank is also known as an over-head tank. Elevated service reservoirs are divided into two parts one part contains the body of the tank and another part contains scaffolding also known as staging of the tank which support the body of the tank. There are different types of elevated tanks based on the scaffolding, structure, and material used to construct the tank. They are

(a) Steel or galvanized iron sheet tank with steel staging for support

(b) Colum made of brick or concrete masonry to support steel tank

(c) Column made of reinforced cement concrete to support reinforced cement concrete tank

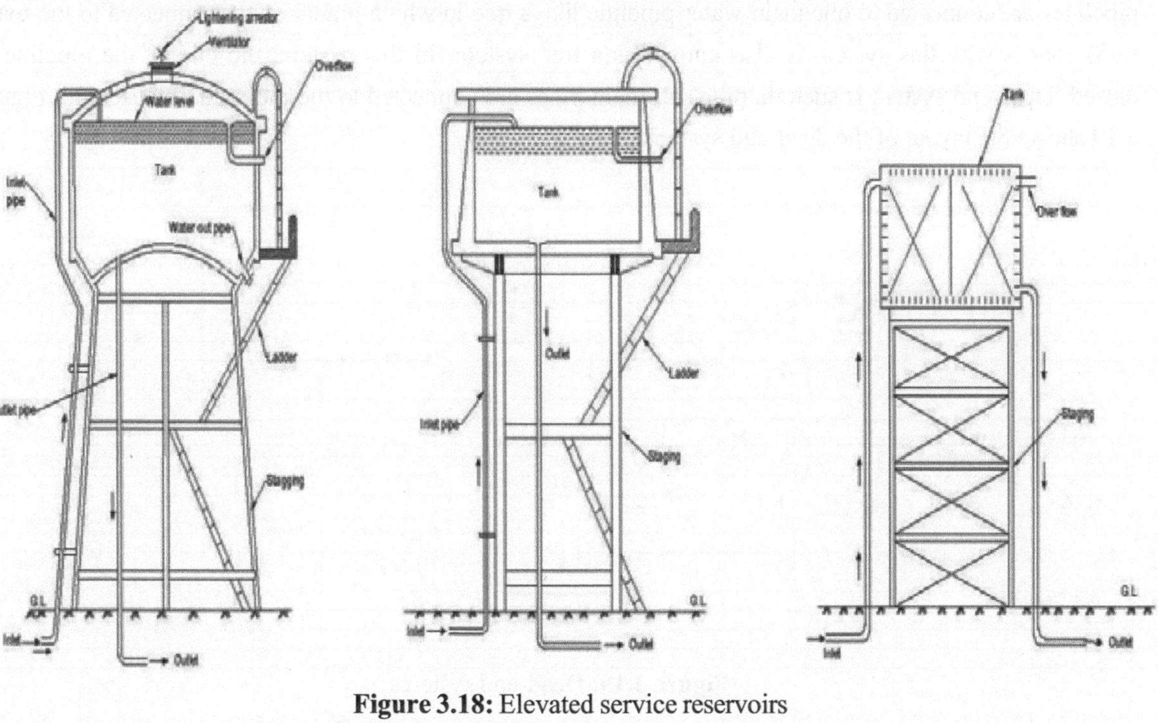

Figure 3.18: Elevated service reservoirs

This type of tank is used for a combined water distribution system for water supply. Water from the treatment plants is stored in this tank and supplied to the individual home. Figure 3.18 shows various types of elevated service tanks used in the water supply. The elevated service reservoir contains all pipe connections such as inlet pipe, outlet pipe, overflow pipe, washout pipe, ventilation, ladder, manhole, gauges, etc. This tank has a meter-wide balcony for inspection and repair work. A floating gauge helps knows the depth of the water in the tank by outside. There is an automatic device installed to stop the pump when tank is full.

3.2.3 Layout of distribution of water

Water distribution system pipeline are laid underground below the road pavements and they generally follows the layout used for the road pavement. They are following systems for laying water distribution pipelines in an area:

1) Dead-end system
2) Grid-iron system
3) Circular system
4) Radial system

This layout systems are explained in the below-mentioned section with their advantage and disadvantages and their suitability.

3.2.3.1 Dead-end system

In this type of distribution of water, the pipelines are laid in such a way that sub-main water supply pipelines are connected to one main water pipeline like a tree in which branches are connected to the main trunk that is why this system is also known as a tree system. In this system, the end of the pipeline is closed. Dead end system is such that the sub-main pipes are connected to the individual household. Figure 3.19 shows the layout of the dead-end system.

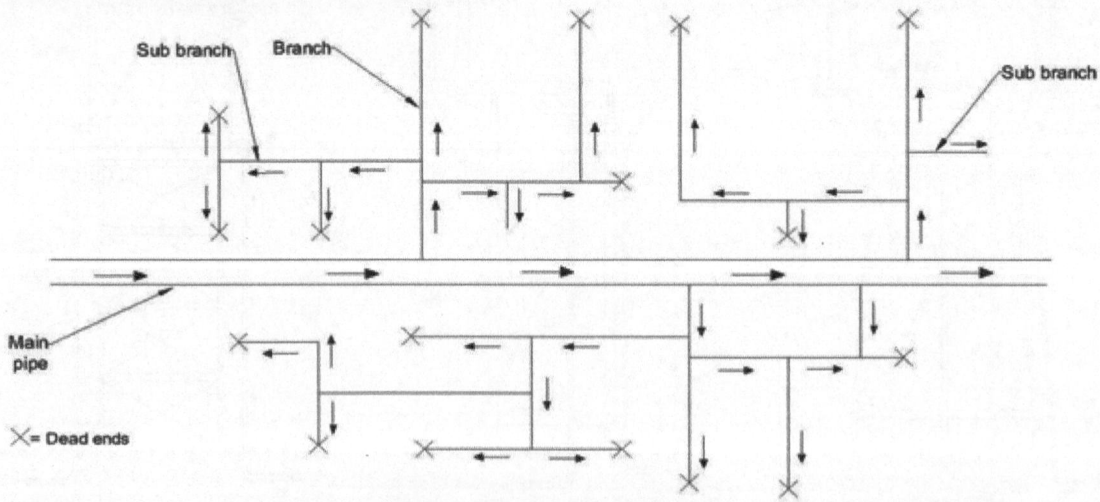

Figure 3.19: Dead-end systems

This system of water distribution is used in old cities or irregular developed settlement of inhabitants and unplanned road in haphazard ways. In this system, the main water pipeline is laid along the main road and branches and sub-branches are taken from this main pipeline wherever the connection is needed which results in the formation of a dead end as can be seen in figure 3.19.

The advantages and disadvantages of this system are discussed below

a) Advantages

i) Less number of gate valves are required in this system

ii) In this system it is easy to determine discharge and pressure at various points in the pipeline
iii) The cost of installing this system is cheap and easily expand
iv) Laying of the pipeline is simple and easy
v) The pipeline length required in this system is shorter length
vi) Inspection of this system pipeline is simple

b) Disadvantages

i) As water reach to particular area through one single main line if there is any repair or maintenance required in particular line then water supply of that particular are will affected and it cause problem to the individual customer.
ii) In this system there are a larger number of dead ends where the water is stagnant and do not circulate. This stagnant water can cause contaminant of water so therefore to remove this stagnant water gate vale is required at every dead end which results in wastage of water.
iii) In case of fire there is a limited supply of water through this system as water flows only in one direction through one pipeline.

3.2.3.2 Grid-iron system

Grid iron system is an improved and improvised form of dead end system. In this system all the main and sub main branches are interconnected to each other as shown in figure 3.20. This type of system can be seen in well planned town where all the major roads and sub roads are made in grid pattern. So, the grid iron pipes can be easily laid in this town under the road. The example of well- planned city such as Chandigarh where the grids iron system of water distribution is laid. The dead end system can be converted to the grid iron system by connected two dead ends to each other. Gate valves are installed at each junction of water pipelines to control the flow of water. The advantages and disadvantages of this system are discussed below.

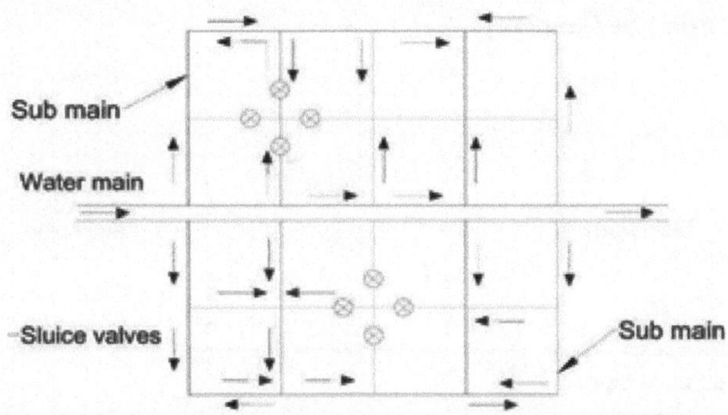

Figure 3.20: Grid-iron system

a) Advantages

i) In this system the water at a point can be reached through different ways so lesser diameter pipe is required and there is the reduction in size due to decrease in friction loss.

ii) The water pressure at different points is same hence head loss will be less.

iii) While repairing and maintenance work is required in a particular section the water has to be diverted for that particular section.

iv) This system do not contains dead end and water is always in circulation which make them free from any contamination.

v) In emergency need and case of fire more water can be diverted by different paths by controlling the flow using a gate valve.

b) Disadvantages

i) In this system there is required a larger number of gate valves and the length of pipe required is more.

ii) The cost of construction is higher.

iii) This system cannot be used in irregularly unplanned towns

iv) It is a difficult and longer process to calculate discharge and pressure accurately in a water pipeline at various points in this method. Required skilled labour and experts to design this system

3.2.3.3 Circular system

This system is also known as a ring system as in this system a circular or rectangular shape main water pipeline periphery is laid in a closed loop and covers the area which has to be served as shown in figure 3.21. In this system, the main pipeline is laid at the outer periphery making a boundary of that area in which water has to be supplied the sub main and branches are connected to the main pipeline to distribute water to individual households. No dead end is formed in this system and water is always remaining in circulation. Water pressure is the same at different points of main and sub-main pipelines. The advantages and disadvantages of this system are discussed below.

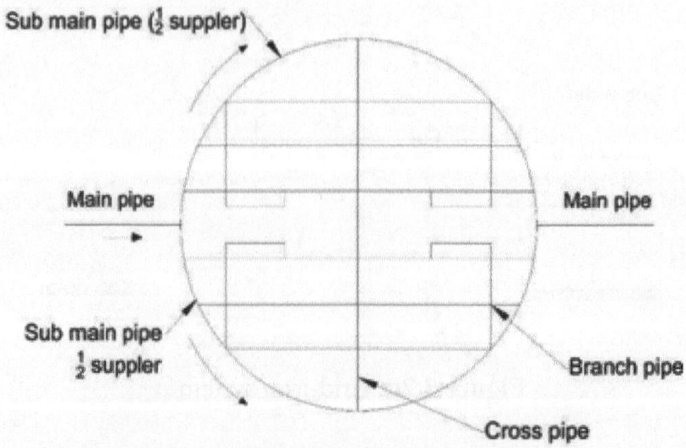

Figure 3.21: Circular or ring system

a) Advantages

i) In this system there is no dead end water always remains in circulation.

ii) The water main pipe line is laid at the periphery of the area which makes same water pressure at different points

iii) During repair and maintenance water is available by the other side

b) Disadvantages

i) In this system there is required a larger number of gate valves and other connection fixtures to control flow of water.

ii) This system requires larger length pipeline as the main line is to be laid at the periphery of the area.

iii) It is costly to install this system.

3.2.3.4 Radial system

This system is the reverse of the circular system as in this system the main water distribution is at the center of the area and from there the water is distributed to individual household using sub main and branch pipelines. This type of system is generally applied in areas which are having radially road network at different centers of the city. In this system, the water from the main pipeline is pumped to different city service reservoirs such as A, B, C, and D as shown in figure 3.22. This service reservoir supplies the water to sub main pipeline which distributes water to the individual household. Different service reservoir are interconnected to each other so that when repairing occurred in one service reservoir the water from other service reservoir can be supplied. The advantages and disadvantages of this system are discussed below.

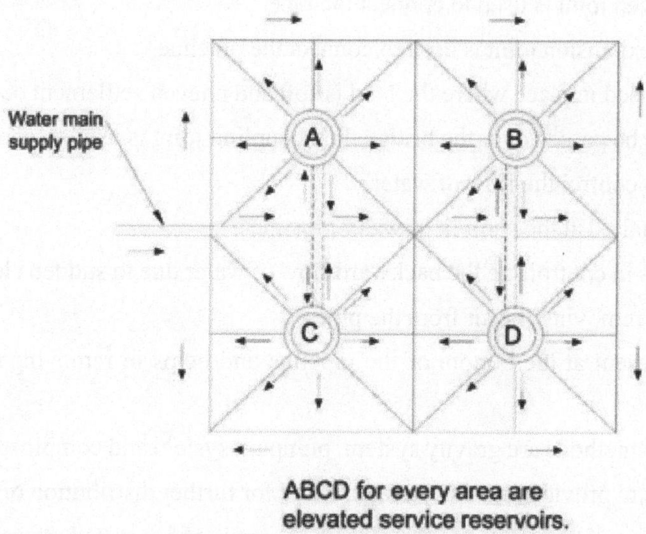

Figure 3.22: Radial system

a) Advantages

i) In this system water pressure remains high and water distribution take place very efficiently.

ii) The calculation of water discharge and design is simple and easy

iii) This system is suitable for any isolated area of a city

iv) In this system there is no dead end and water remains in circulation

v) The distribution tank of each area is also served as a service reservoir of that area.

b) Disadvantages

i) This system is only situated in areas that have radial road network

ii) This system is expensive as a separate distribution tank has to be made for each sub-area.

UNIT SUMMARY

- The water using conveyance transport through gravity or by pressure.
- In gravity conveyance the water flows due to gravitational force.
- Pressure conveyance is closed pipe in which water flow under pressure.
- Cast iron pipes are widely used in India for water conveyance.
- Steel pipes are used for main water supply, inverted syphon and where water is to pass through high pressure.
- *Galvanized pipes are used in household fittings using screwed and socket joint*
- Reinforced cement concrete pipes can take compressive load and do not collapse due to heavy traffic load.
- Plastic pipes are now days very common for house hold fittings.
- Socket and spigot joint are joint by skilled labour.
- In steel pipes flanged joint is used to connect the pipe.
- In cast iron pipes expansion joint is used to connect the pipeline.
- Flexible joint are used in place where the land is soft and uneven settlement occur.
- When pipes are to be passed over the bridge then coupling joint is used to connect the water pipeline.
- Valves are used to control the flow of water.
- Gate valve are installed at the summit of water pipeline
- Reflux valve helps in controlling the backward flow of water due to sudden closer of pump
- Air valve helps in removing the air from the pipes.
- Scour valve is present at the bottom of the pipeline and helps in removing the impurities from the pipe line.
- Water distribution methods are gravity system, pumping system and combined system.
- Service reservoir are provide to collect treated water for further distribution of water
- Service reservoir are of two types gravity service reservoir and elevated service reservoir
- Elevated service reservoir has two parts one is body of the tank and other is staging for support of tank.
- In dead end system the water get stuck at the end of the pipe line
- Grid iron system there is no dead end the water always remain in circulation.

EXERCISES

Multiple Choice Questions

1. Which of the following statement is right related to grid iron distribution system
   (a) Best situated foe well planned cities (b) lower number of gate valve is required
   (c) Construction is easy (d) All of the above
2. In which distribution system the treated water flow under gravity
   (a) Gravity system (b) Pressure system
   (c) Pumping system (d) None of these
3. Which valve is used to stop the flow of water for repairing and maintenance
   (a) Air relief valve (b) Pressure relief valve
   (c) Gate valve (d) None
4. Gate valve is made of which material
   (a) Reinforced cement concrete (b) Cement concrete
   (c) Cast iron (d) All of the above
5. Which valve allow water to flow in one direction
   (a) Gate valve (b) Reflux valve
   (c) Air relief valve (d) Pressure relief valve
6. The location at which air relief valve provide in pipeline
   (a) At valley (b) At summit
   (c) At joints (d) None of these
7. Which of the following is not a method of layout of distribution system
   (a) Dead end system (b) Grid iron system
   (c) Rng system (d) Pressure system
8. Which of the distribution system layout is used of irregular cities:
   (a) Dead end system (b) Grid iron system
   (c) Both of these (d) Pressure system
9. The amount of lead required to join 150 mm diameter cast iron pipe using socket and spiogot joint
   (a) 5 kg (b) 4 kg
   (c) 3.5 kg (d) All of the above
10. Which of the joint is used in place where temperature changes
    (a) Expansion joint (b) Flanged joint
    (c) socket and spigot joint (d) All of the above
11. How much pressure does asbestos cement pipe can handle?
    (a) 35 Kg/cm^2 (b) 45 Kg/cm^2
    (c) 25 Kg/cm^2 (d) None
12. Which valve is also known as washout valve
    (a) Scour valve (b) Gate valve
    (c) Reflux valve (d) Air relief valve

Answers of Multiple Choice Questions

1. (a), 2. (a), 3. (c), 4. (c), 5. (b), 6. (b), 7. (d), 8. (a), 9. (c) 10. (a) 11. (c) 12. (a)

Short and Long Answer Type Questions

1. Describe the name and properties of pipes used in water supply.
2. Write a short note on cast-iron pipes and galvanized iron pipe.
3. Which pipe would you use for rising main and internal water system
4. Why, where and under what condition are joints in pipes installed?
5. Describe the following with diagram.
   a) Socket and spiogot b) Flanged joint c) Expansion joint d) Thread socket joint
6. Explain with diagram joints used in galvanised iron.
7. Why are valves installed on the pipeline?
8. Describe gate valve and reflux valve with diagram
9. Explain air relief valve with neat diagram
10. Describe with neat diagram how are collar joint installed on concrete pipes?
11. You are coming towards down slope while installing a pipeline on sloping ground. Explain where you will place the socket end of the pipe.
12. In the water distribution system, why there is a need for water storage?
13. Explain the importance of elevated service reservoir.
14. Explain the difference between gravity distribution system and pressure distribution system.
15. Explain the dead end layout of water distribution with diagram.
16. Write short note on radial layout and circular layout of distribution system
17. Write advantages and disadvantages of grid iron system.

REFERENCES AND SUGGESTED READINGS

1. Sharma S.C, Environmental Engineering, Khanna Publishing House, New Delhi
2. Garg, S.K., Environmental Engineering Vol. I and Vol. II, Khanna Publishers
3. Birdie, G. S. and Birdie, J. S.Water Supply and Sanitary Engineering, Dhanpat Rai
4. Gupta, O.P., Elements of Environmental Pollution Control, Khanna Publishing House, Delhi
5. Rao, C.S., Environmental Pollution Control Engineering, New Age International.
6. IS Code 1536-1976
7. IS Code 458-2021
8. IS Code 3076:1985 (Re 2003)
9. IS Code 4984:1995 (Re 2002)
10. IS Code 4985:2000
11. Punmia, B C, Environmental Engineering, vol. I and II, Laxmi Publishers
12. Basak N N, Environmental Engineering, McGraw Hill Publishers.

4 Domestic Sewage and System of Sewerages

UNIT SPECIFICS

Through this unit we have discussed the following aspects:

- *To understand various components of building sanitation*
- *Understand various types of sanitary fittings and their uses*
- *Overview of the plumbing system*
- *Overview of sewerage systems*
- *Discussion on sewer laying and testing*
- *Introduction of manhole*

To help the students in the visualization of the content and to enhance their practical knowledge, the figures are provided in 2D. The content in this unit provides practical knowledge and will help the students in decision-making during the fieldwork.

This unit contains short and long answer-type questions along with multiple choice questions, a list of references, and suggested reading so that one can go through them for practice. Some QR codes are given which can be scanned for more information on various topics of interest and to get extra knowledge.

RATIONALE

This unit on the domestic sewage and system of sewerage helps the students to develop an idea about the building sanitation and sewerage system. It explains the principles required for design of building drainage. The various terms used in building sanitation are discussed. A brief discussion about building sanitary fittings is provided. The various types of traps are also discussed and an introduction about inspection and junction chamber is given. The content covered in this unit is important to understand the process of building drainage system.

The knowledge of building sanitation, sewerage system and sewer appurtenances are essential for civil engineering students. The students can apply the knowledge of for designing the building sanitation and drainage. The knowledge gained in this unit will help the students to suitable fittings and traps for different sanitation fittings. The students can apply their knowledge in the selection and implementation of suitable system of sewerage. The concepts in this unit will help the student in effective supervision of construction works of the building drainage.

PRE-REQUISITES

A basic knowledge of building components is required.

UNIT OUTCOMES

The list of outcomes of this unit is as follows:

U4-O1: *To explain the process of the building sanitation.*

U4-O2: *To understand the process of system of plumbing.*

U4-O3: *To realize the suitability of different building sanitary fittings for the different operation.*

U4-O4: *To determine the function and suitability of different types of sewerage system.*

U4-O5: *To propose a suitable design principle for building drainage.*

Unit-4 Outcomes	EXPECTED MAPPING WITH COURSE OUTCOMES (1- Weak Correlation; 2- Medium correlation; 3- Strong Correlation)				
	CO-1	CO-2	CO-3	CO-4	CO-5
U4-O1	-	-	-	-	1
U4-O2	-	-	1	-	1
U4-O3	-	-	-	-	-
U4-O4	-	-	1	-	-
U4-O5	-	1	-	-	2

4.1 Building sanitation: Necessity of sanitation

Nowadays, most of the peoples are moving to cities and town from the village to live a modern and to increase the living standard which results in over population of the town. This overburden of town leads to turn the pure and clean environment to polluted environment. Sanitation department dealt with this polluted environment so that clean and pure environment condition will offer to the human beings. As the population is increasing in the towns the older methods which are time consuming are discard and with the advancement in engineering and science many new sanitation techniques are developed and adopted worldwide to dispose the fecal matter and urine. For proper sanitation of the buildings various sanitation fittings and pipes are properly installed according to their location and use. In sanitation the proper drainage and sanitation fitting and disposal of sewage from the city is covered.

4.1.1 Necessity to treat domestic sewage

Domestic sewage includes wastewater from the toilets, kitchen, washing clothes, etc. Nature can treat pollution but with the increase in pollution, the sewage is also increased considerably resulting in the development of techniques for sewage treatment. In sewage treatment, the pollution and sewage are reduced to an amount that nature can handle. If there is no domestic sewage treatment plant then there occurs nuisance all around and human beings cannot leave in the surrounding. In domestic sewage treatment, the treatment occurs in two parts. In first part is known as primary treatment in which about 65% of suspended particles are removed from the wastewater and the other is secondary treatment in which all organic and inorganic pollution is removed by using various biological mechanisms such as sequential batch reactors, membrane biofilms, etc. after the treatment the treated effluent from the wastewater treatment plant is discharged to use in irrigation use or discharge into the rivers.

4.1.2 Definitions

(a) **Sewage:** Sewage is defined as wastewater containing waste from human excreta, urine, industrial wastewater, commercial wastewater, household waste from the kitchen, bathroom, and water from the runoff during a storm. Sewage contains suspended and dissolved impurities of organic and inorganic matter.

(b) **Sullage:** Sullage is a type of wastewater that includes wastewater from household activities from the kitchen and bathroom except waste related to human excreta and urine. It is also known as grey water.

(c) **Types of sewage:** Sewage is classified into three types. They are:

i) **Domestic sewage:** Domestic sewage includes the wastewater that comes from the bathroom room including the flushing system, clothes washing, and kitchen including water from washing utensils from residential households. In this sewage the water contains about 99.9%. This sewage flows in closed pipes as it begins to smell and odor after some time.

ii) **Industrial sewage:** Industrial sewage includes the wastewater from different industrial processes, factories, and workshops. The water used for running the machines contains various types of dirt. Industrial sewage contains various harmful chemicals and metals which require specific treatment to remove. So industrial sewage is generally treated separately from domestic sewage.

iii) **Strom Water:** when rain takes place in a city or town some part of the water penetrates the ground and the remaining water flows on the surface of the land and gets collected to the open drain. This remaining water on the surface of the land is known as stormwater or run-off water. Strom water also includes water from the rooftop of the household if discharged into the open drain.

4.1.3 Definition of the terms related to Building Sanitation

(1) Rainwater pipe: Rainwater pipes are installed to bring the rainwater from the roof to the ground. They are installed vertically in the direction along the external wall of the building. It is also known as a downpipe. These pipes are made up of asbestos or cement. Their diameter is kept at a minimum of 150 mm. Iron mesh is installed at the opening of the pipe so that any garbage or stone pipe does not enter the pipe, if they enter they can block the pipe. These pipes are installed in such a way that for every 30 m^2 of roof area a pipe of 150 mm is installed to bring the rainwater down to the ground. These pipes do not enter the direction of the sewer line as they can bring the contaminated gases from the sewer to the buildings so a gully trap is provided at the bottom of the water pipe as seen in figure 4.1.

(2) Soil Pipe: This pipe is used to carry the waste/urine from the toilet to the domestic sewer line. This pipe is made up of cast iron and stoneware material. The minimum diameter of this pipe is kept at 100 mm. The joint used to connect the soil pipe is the socket and spigot joint. This pipe is installed on the outer wall to bring down sewage from the upper floor. At the top end of the pipe, a cowl is installed as can see in figure 4.1. There is no gully trap installed at the bottom end of the pipe. Soil pipe is connected to the manhole at the bottom so that is there is any chance of blocking in soil pipe it can be cleaned using manhole.

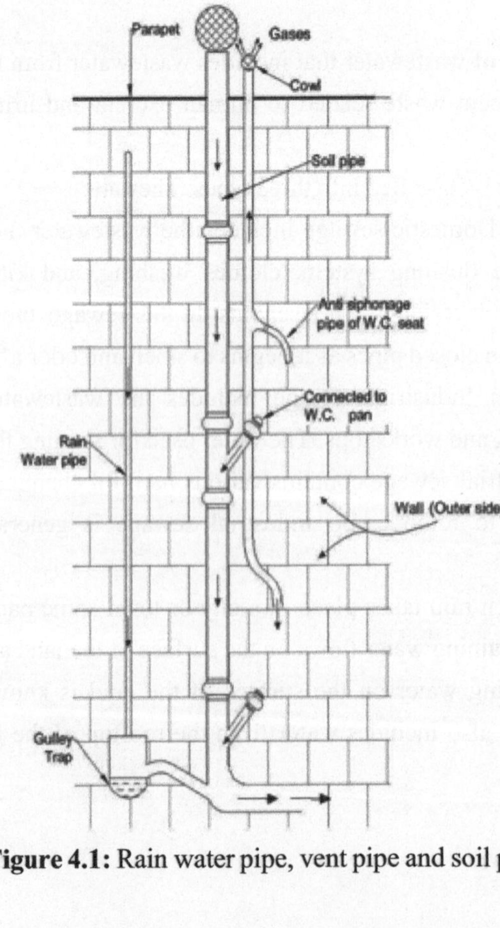

Figure 4.1: Rain water pipe, vent pipe and soil pipe

(3) Sullage pipe: Sullage pipe is a type of pipe that carries waste from the bathroom, kitchen, wash basin, and washing of clothes. The waste from flushing water is not carried in this pipe. A gully trap is provided at the bottom of the sullage pipe before connecting to the domestic sewer line. The diameter of the sullage pipe should be kept at a minimum of 75 mm.

(4) Vent Pipe: In the flushing system when a sufficient amount of water is released during flushing the water flows suddenly then the stagnant water in the traps also escapes through the soil pipe which occurs due to the creation of a partial vacuum. In a multi-storied building, all the flushing system latrines are connected to the same soil pipe and when the flushing system comes down rapidly it removes the air present in the pipes and creates a partial vacuum. Due to this sudden flow of water, the water seal present in the traps of the lower floor breaks down. Due to this, the contaminated gases come start to the lower floor and foul smell and odor start from latrines. This whole action is known as inverted siphonage. Vent pipes are installed to prevent this siphon action in the building and a smaller diameter (around 50 mm) pipe is installed. A vent pipe is connected to the trap of the toilet from the top. Vent pipe also helps in releasing the contaminated gases collected in sewer lines. An iron cowl is installed at the top end of the pipe to prevent birds from entering the pipeline. This pipe is kept about 150 cm above the roof. Figure 4.1 shows the arrangement of the vent pipe.

4.1.4 Building sanitary fittings

Different bathroom fittings such as water closets, cisterns, wash basins, sinks, and urinals are installed in the toilets in the proper place for hand-washing, bathing, etc. are known as building sanitary fittings. These different fittings are made up of different materials such as china clay, plastics, glazed clay, brass, cast iron, etc. Building sanitary fittings are generally kept near an outer wall so that the least pipe length required for connection and availability of natural light and fresh air is easy. Various building sanitary fittings are explained in the below-mentioned section.

4.1.4.1 Water closet

The water closet is a plumbing system installed in latrines to receive human excreta and it is directly connected to soil pipe using a trap. The water closet is installed near the outer wall to make connection easy. Sometimes water closet refers to the entire toilet in place to only a few sanitary fittings which are installed in the toilet.

Different water closet system can be addressed in terms of economy, location, etc. They are listed as follows:

1. Indian-type water closet
2. European-type water closet

These two types of water closets are explained below.

1. Indian-type water closet: In this type of water closet the trap and the squatting pan are two different items that are connected and kept below the floor level. In this water closet, the seat is kept a minimum of

450 mm long and the depth of the seat and trap is kept a minimum of 400 mm. In this P-trap or S-trap is used which is connected with the soil pipe. The material used for the seat is vitreous china. A hollow box-type flushing rim is made at the top of the toilet seat. This hollow box has a hole at the bottom which is used to flush the water. Indian type of water closets is of the following types:

i) **Long Type Water Closet Seat:** Long type seat has a seat size that varies from 450 mm to 680 mm. The largest size seat size 680 mm is not used. Two footrests are placed next to the seat on each side. The trap is connected to the bottom of the seat to form a water seal which helps in preventing the contaminated gases from entering the chamber. The trap is connected with the vent pipe and soil pipe. A hollow rim is installed above the seat in which holes is there at the bottom to which pipe is connected to the seat. The human excreta do not fall directly into the trap instead it falls on the seat. The hollow flushing system helps in moving the excreta from the seat to the soil pipe. If the flushing system is not working properly then the excreta will not flush properly and a foul smell will be left. These water closets require around 10 liters of water for flushing the excreta. A typical section of a long type of India water closet is seen in figure 4.2.

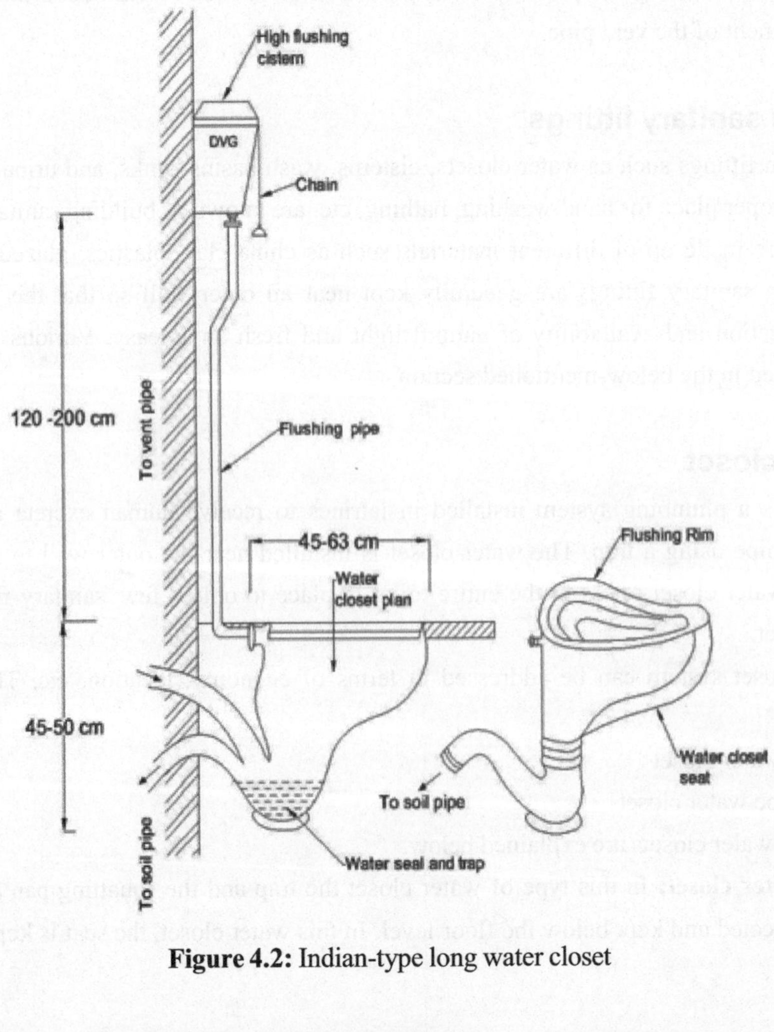

Figure 4.2: Indian-type long water closet

ii) **Orissa Pattern water closet seat:** The length of this seat varies from 580 mm to 680 mm. In this pattern, the seat is attached to the foot rest as seen in figure 4.3. This is the most common type of seat used in Indian households. A separate flushing system is attached to the end of the seat to move the human excreta to the soil pipe.

iii) **Rural seat:** This seat is mostly used in rural areas because they require less amount of water to move the excreta as this seat does not have any hollow to attach the flushing system. Water is poured from the above to move the stool from the squatting pan. This seat has a septic tank at the bottom to collect the sewage. This seat has a maximum length of 450 mm. Figure 4.4 shows the rural type seat.

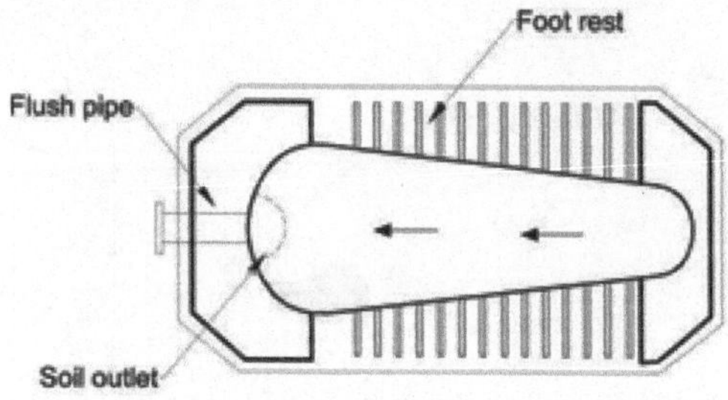

Figure 4.3: Orissa pattern water closet

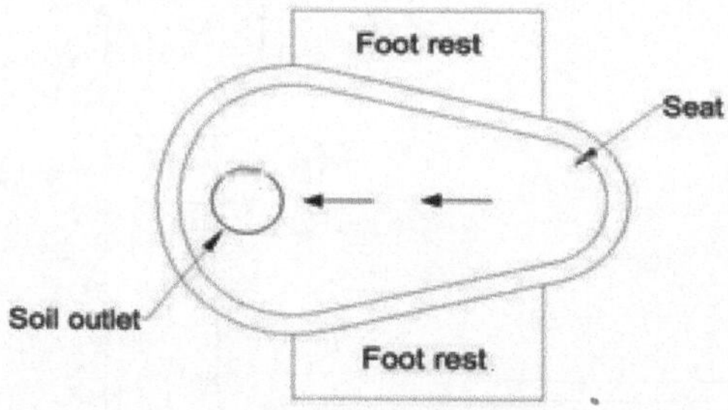

Figure 4.4: Rural seat

2. European-type water closet: This type of water closet is mostly used in Western countries and India in high-class residential buildings or hotels. However with the modernization in Indian households, their use has increased. This type of water closet is installed above the floor on the pedestal so, it is also known as a pedestal seat. In this water closet, the seat and trap is molded as one unit. This seat takes less space as compared to an Indian-style seat. The plastic rim is attached to the seat on which the person sits. It has a plastic lid cover to cover the seat when not in use. This type of water closet has a vertical back and the outlet hole is placed in such a way that human excreta does not stay on the seat. Figure 4.5 shows the European water closet seat.

The flushing system used in this closet is placed near the seat and can be used while sitting on the seat. Two types of traps (P trap or S trap) are used in this seat depending on the location of fitting of the seat on the floor or in the wall. The seat length varies from 480 mm to 630 mm and the height of the seat varies from 350 mm to 400 mm. European-type water closets are of two types:

i) Wash-down type pan: The rims provided for flushing have a larger width and the water seal provided as a trap has a depth of 50 mm. In this, there is an inlet pipe which is connecting to the flush. Human excreta fall directly into the water seal and trap as can be seen in figure 4.6. There is only one trap in this type of seat.

ii) Syphon-type pan: This type of water closet has two traps connected to the seat and soil pipe as can be seen in figure 4.7. The bend between the two traps is connected to the flushing system by a low-diameter pipe. When we flush the water drops suddenly from the flush system and the air that is present in the flush pipe is drawn into the smaller diameter pipe which creates partial pressure and the conditions of siphon occur. This siphon action helps in the quick discharge of sewage to soil pipes.

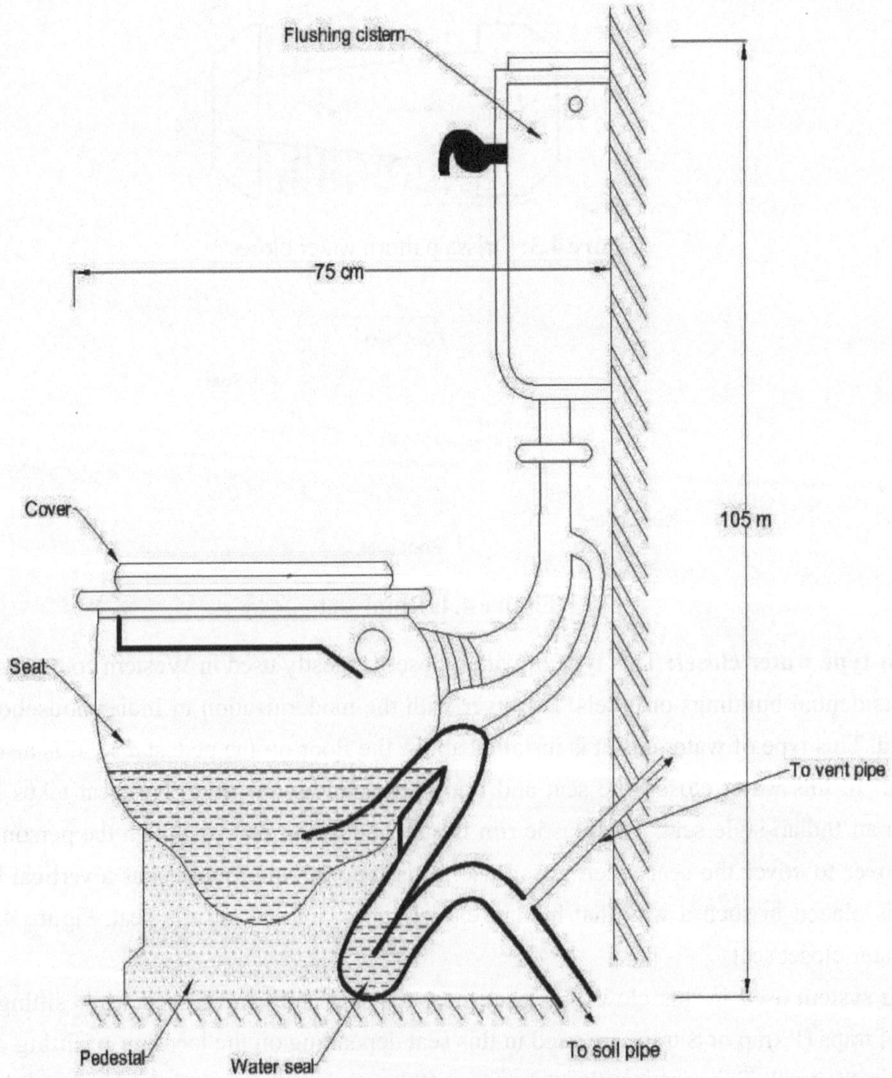

Figure 4.5: European-type water closet

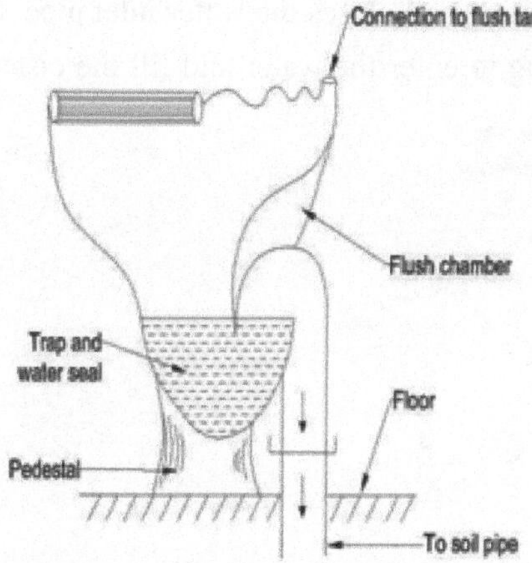

Figure 4.6: Wash down type pan

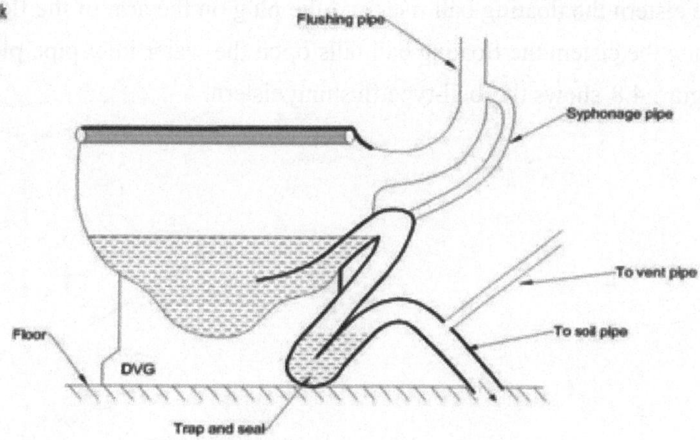

Figure 4.7: Syphon type pan

4.1.4.2 Flushing cistern

A flushing cistern is a type of apparatus through which a known quantity of water is discharged through pressure to remove the stool from the pan of the water closet or to remove the urinals. They are installed above the seat. Due to their location above the seat, they can be classified as high-level cisterns which are installed at a minimum height of 125 cm above the seat and another type is a low-level cistern which has a minimum height of 30 cm. Low-level cistern is used in European type water closet while in Indian style water closet, both high level and low- level cistern can be used. A high-level cistern is operated by a hanging chain while in low level cistern lever mechanism is used to operate. Different materials such as cast iron, glazed vitreous ware, porcelain enamel, etc. are used to manufacture flushing cisterns. Nowadays plastic flushing cisterns are commonly used. IS 774-2004 which is related to the design and construction of a flushing cistern in India said that the discharge rate of a flushing cistern should be 5 liters in 3 seconds and 6 seconds it should discharge 10 liters.

Flushing Cistern can be classified into three types based on structure. They are explained in the below-mentioned section.

(a) **Bell Type Cistern:** Bell-type flushing cisterns do not have any type of valve and they are generally made up of cast iron which has a capacity of around 10 liters to 15 liters. In this flushing cistern, the center is kept a little bit lower than the other side and the outlet pipe is deep inside the cast iron box. A chain is connected to the bell with the help of a lever arm. There is a hole in the bell through which water is passed down when the chain is pulled by the jerk. Due to this jerk, the water through the bell moves down to the outlet pipe and the air present in the pipes moves downward direction causing a partial vacuum in the bell which triggers the symphonic action. Due to this symphonic action, the water moves rapidly through the outlet pipe and flush the toilet. To create this symphonic action the chain should be pulled with jerk.

The floating ball is attached to the water inlet pipe having a plug at the top of the arm of the floating ball. The floating ball controls the water level in the flushing cistern. When the water reaches a specific level in the cistern the floating ball rises and the plug on the arm of the floating ball closes the water inlet pipe. On using the cistern the floating ball falls open the water inlet pipe plug to enter the water and fill the cistern. Figure 4.8 shows the bell-type flushing cistern.

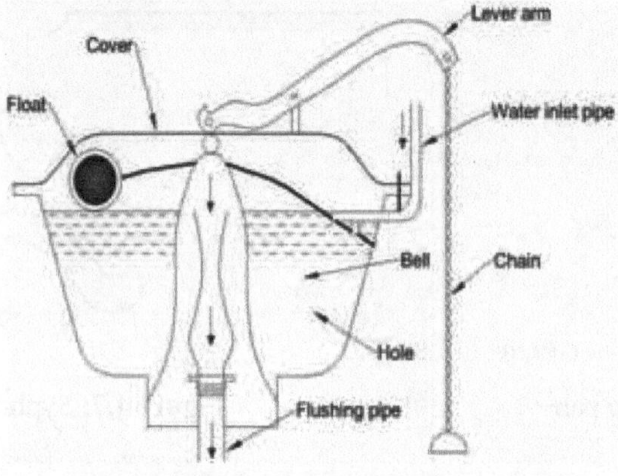

Figure 4.8: Bell type flushing cistern

An overflow, pipe is also provided in this type of flushing cistern in case the floating ball strikes then over overflow pipe will release the extra water. Water inlet pipes have a diameter of 15 mm and the outlet overflow pipe has a diameter of 20 mm. Outlet pipe from the cistern has a diameter of 30 mm. This cistern is installed at a minimum height of 125 cm from the seat to work properly. Bell type of flushing cistern discharges the same amount of water whenever you pull the chain but in the case of urinals a small amount of water is required and in places where there is a shortage of water this type of flushing cistern is not used.

(b) **Flat-bottom type flushing cistern:** This type of flushing cistern has valves to control the flow of water. In this cistern, the outlet pipe has a U-shaped bend at the upper end as seen in figure 4.9. The lower side pipe of the U-type pipe has a cylinder. There is a valve in the shape of a disc is attached to this cylinder bottom. This disc-shaped valve is attached with the help of a chain to the lever arm and the lever arm is attached to another chain which is used to pull the lever as can be seen in figure 4.9. When we pull the chain the disc valve rises and lets the water flow down through the shaped pipe.

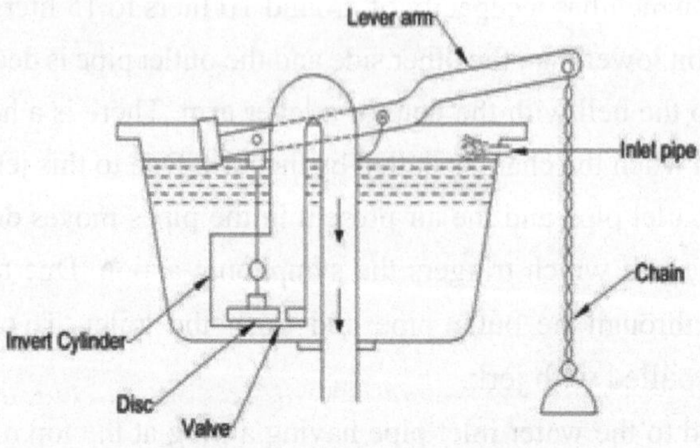

Figure 4.9: Flat bottom type flushing cistern

(c) **Automatic Flushing type:** In this tank, the water is filled at a specific level with a fixed rate and after reaching that level the water automatically flushes causing the symphonic action. This type of flushing cistern is used for urinals and has a capacity of around 5 liters. There is cock on the water inlet pipe which can be adjusted as per the requirement of water and the interval at which the tank is filled. Generally, the time taken to fill the tank is 10 to 15 minutes.

4.1.4.3 Washbasin

Washbasins have vessels and are used to wash hands, mouth, and teeth. The materials used to make the washbasin are vitrified clay, china clay, and glazed stoneware but nowadays they are available in stainless steel, plastic, and aluminum. Wash basin having one or more than one water tap in the middle of the basin through which hot and cold water connection is done. Nowadays a mixture tap is installed in place of two water taps in which either cold, hot, or mixed of both hot and cold water can come as per the requirement of the individual. An outlet pipe is provided at the center of the basin it is covered with iron or steel mesh to protect the pipe from choking by large particles. The trap is provided at the end of the waste pipe. The height of the basin is kept around 800mm from the floor. Based on the type of support the wash basin is used to install them can be classified into two types:

i) **Flatback:** This type of wash basin is installed into the wall by using brackets and they are fixed to the wall as shown in figure 4.10. This wash basin has a flat back but sometimes an angle back is provided to fix the wash basin at the junction of the wall. The size of the basin for flat back varies from 400 to 450 mm by 550 to 650 mm and for angle back, the size varies from 400 to 480 mm by 400 to 600 mm.

ii) **Pedestal:** This type of wash basin is installed on the pedestal which is installed on the floor. Their size also varies from 450 mm to 650 mm. Figure 4.11 shows the pedestal type wash basin.

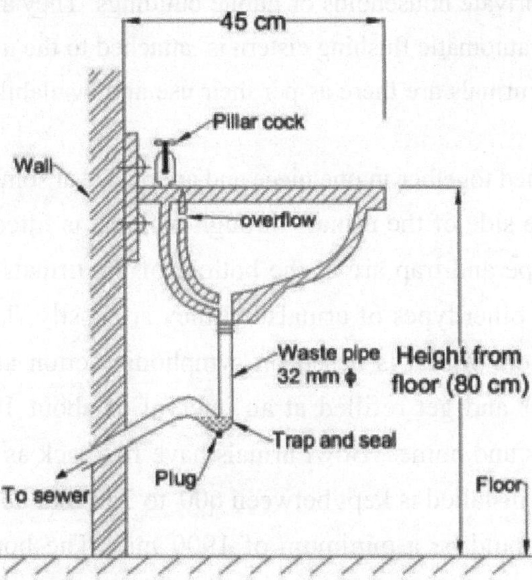

Figure 4.10: Flat back wash basin

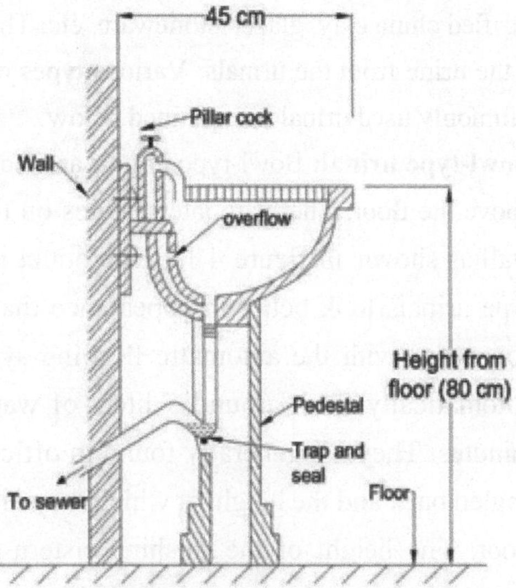

Figure 4.11: Pedestal wash basin

4.1.4.4 Sinks

Sinks are square or rectangular in shape and are used to wash utensils in the kitchen. They are shallow in depth. Waste outlet is provided at the center of the bottom of the vessel. The center of the vessel is kept lower than the edges so that water can be removed easily as kitchen utensils contain food waste which if remain on the vessels can create a foul smell.

There is no rim attached to the sink and they are made up of stainless steel, aluminum, or marble. A minimum height of around 900 mm from the floor is kept while installing the sink. Figure 4.12 shows the sink. The kitchen size is available in different sizes with dimensions varies from length 600 mm to 750 mm, width of 450 mm, and depth of 150 mm to 250 mm. while laboratory sink dimensions vary as length 400 mm to 600 mm, width of 250 mm to 400 mm and depth 150 mm to 250 mm.

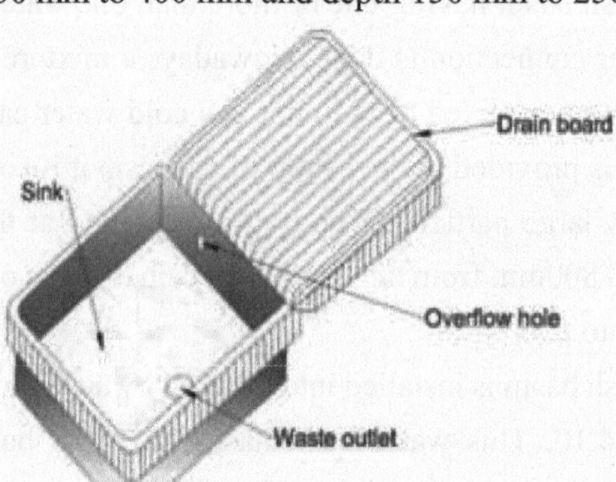

Figure 4.12: Sink

4.1.4.5 Urinals

Urinals are used to urinate in standing positions in private households or public buildings. They are made up of vitrified china clay, glazed stoneware, etc. The automatic flushing cistern is attached to the urinals to remove the urine from the urinals. Various types of urinals are there as per their use and availability. The most commonly used urinal is explained below:

(a) **Bowl-type urinal:** Bowl-type urinals are molded together in one piece and are placed at some height above the floor. There are lateral holes on the side of the urinals through which it is fitted on the wall as shown in figure 4.13. The outlet pipe and trap are at the bottom of the urinals. Bowl-type urinals look better in appearance than other types of urinals but they are costly. They are connected with the automatic flushing system which is based on symphonic action and they automatically flush around 5 liters of water and get refilled at an interval of about 10 to 15 minutes. They are generally found in offices and homes. Bowl urinals have flat back as well as angled back and the height at which they are installed is kept between 600 to 750 mm above the floor. The height of the flushing cistern should be a minimum of 1900 mm. The horizontal spacing between the two urinals is kept around 600 mm.

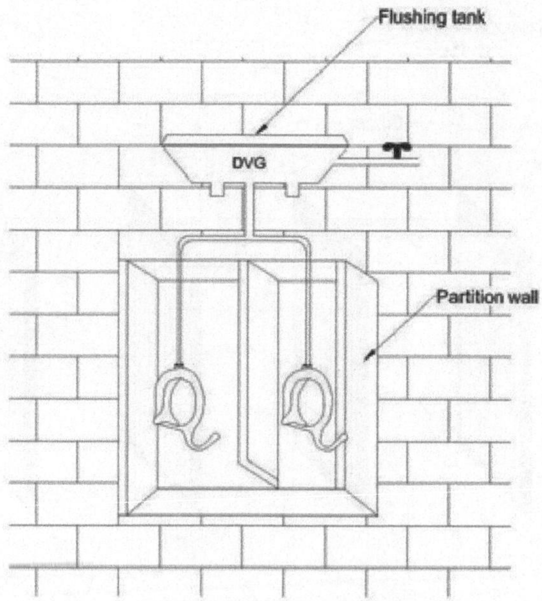

Figure 4.13: Bowl urinal

(b) **Slab and stall-type urinals:** These urinals are placed in places where a large number of crowds visit such as railway stations, cinema halls, large factories, schools, colleges etc. In this type of urinal, there are several compartments are made by placing small curtain walls at some height and urinals are placed on each compartment for urine as shown in figure 4.14. Each compartment of this urinal type has a height of around 1 meter and the spacing between two urinals is kept around 600 mm. The height of the curtain wall is kept at around 750 mm. Glazed tiles are placed on the wall where a person passes urine and this urine is collected on the drain pipe which is laid on the floor. This drain pipe is connected to the soil pipe to carry the urine to the sewage. A flushing tank with a capacity of 10 to 15 liters is attached for flushing.

(c) **Squatting urinals:** They are also known as lady urinals as they are specifically made for the use of ladies. These types of urinals are made in such a way that they can sit and urinate. They are found in high-class buildings. Figure 4.15 shows the lady's urinal. They have dimensions that vary in length from 450 to 600 mm and in width from 300 to 400 mm. Flushing pipes are connected to the flushing cistern.

The manufacturing of urinals is carried out as per the provision given in the Bureau of Indian Standards. IS 771-1979 has given standards for manufacturing of glazed earthenware urinals and IS 2556 (Part 6) -2021 has given standards for vitreous china urinals.

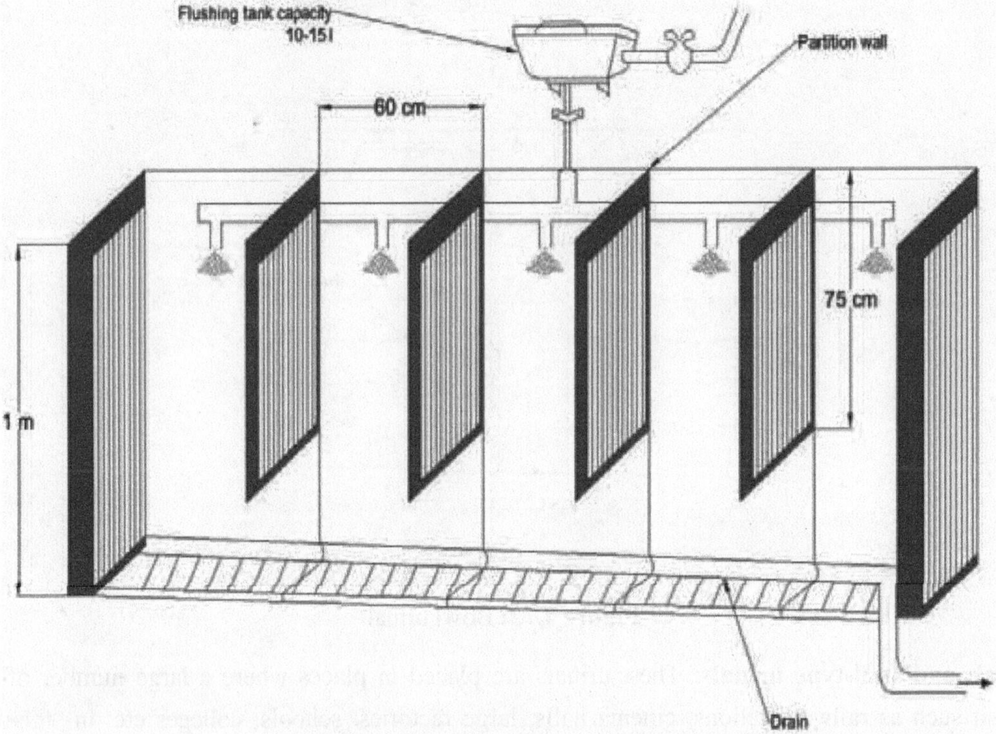

Figure 4.14: Slab and stall-type urinal

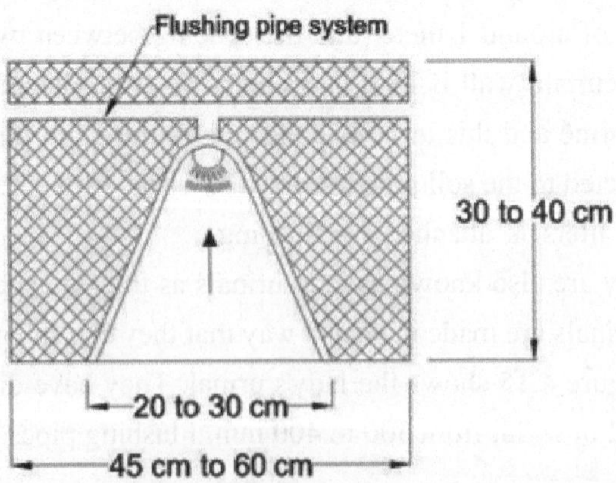

Figure 4.15: Squatting urinal

4.1.5 Traps

Various types of contaminated gases are produced in soil pipes, sewage drains, and waste drains which can infiltrate into the household by these pipes. To stop these contaminated gases from entering the buildings traps are installed. Traps are sanitary fittings that are installed at the end of drainage pipes or sanitary equipment before joining the pipes to soil pipes or sewage drains to prevent foul gases from entering the buildings. Traps help in achieving this by maintaining the water seal between the sanitary fitting and soil pipe.

Trap efficiency depends on the depth of the water seal they produce between the soil pipe and sanitary fitting. Traps are generally u-shaped bend pipes which is filled with water up to a certain depth. To maintain the effectiveness of the trap a water depth of 50 mm is required but depth varies from 25 mm to 75 mm.

4.1.5.1 Types of Traps

Traps can be classified into different types based on their shape and use. Classification based on shapes is explained in the below section and the types of traps based on uses is explained.

Traps classification based on shapes are:

i. P trap
ii. Q trap
iii. S trap
iv. V trap
v. D trap
vi. Anti-siphon trap

The names of the traps are given as per their design shape which can be seen in figure 4.16 [(i) to (vi)]. The first three traps i.e. P, Q, and S traps are the most common types of traps used in sanitary fittings in toilets, bathrooms, and sinks. These traps consist of u shaped pipe which helps in maintain the water seal and prevents the leakage of foul gas. V trap is applied when there is horizontal flow in the pipeline. The outlet end of the trap is somewhat larger in diameter than the inlet end to let the flush water exit well. D trap has higher water seal depth as compared to other traps and has an outlet end bigger than the inlet end which helps in reducing the momentum of discharge.

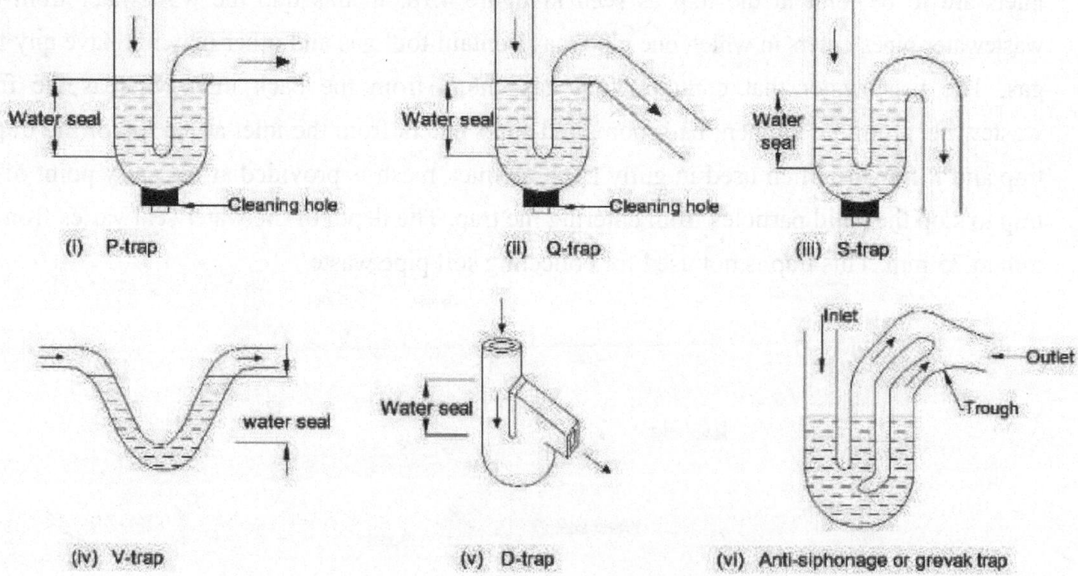

Figure 4.16: Different types of traps

The anti-siphon trap helps in maintaining the siphon action in the traps and helps in maintaining the water seals. This trap is also known as a great trap. While using this trap there is no need to provide a separate mechanism for siphon action.

Traps classification based on uses are:

(a) **Floor trap:** Floor traps are provided where wastewater is collected from the bathroom, kitchen, and sinks. In these traps generally, P and S trap shape trap is used. The depth of the water seal in this trap is between 35 mm to 50 mm. Thick cast iron or galvanized iron and stainless-steel mesh is provided at the entry to stop the entry of garbage or any solid particle that can block the trap. There is a hinge is provided on the mesh to lift up the cover and clean the trap. Figure 4.17 shows the floor trap. They are also known as nahani traps. The inlet diameter of the trap is about 150 mm.

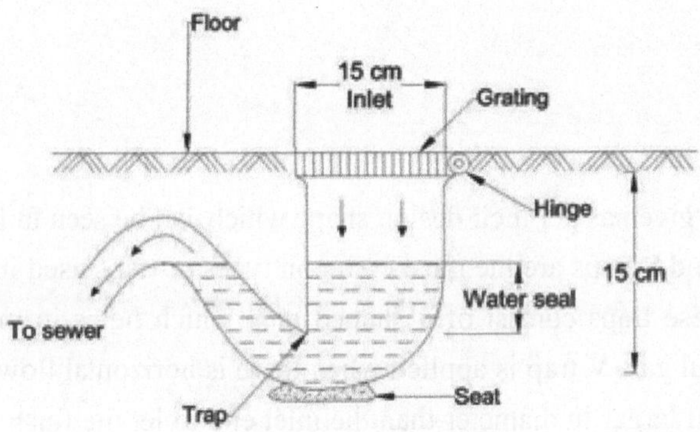

Figure 4.17: Floor trap

(b) **Gully trap:** This type of trap is provided at the interception of a room or where two or more two inlets are to be joint in the trap as seen in figure 4.18. In this trap the wastewater from two wastewater pipes enters in which one pipe may contain foul gas and other may not have any foul gas. The wastewater that contains foul gas enters from the back inlet whereas the fresh wastewater from the kitchen, bathroom, and sinks enters from the inlet at the top of the trap. S trap and P trap are often used in gully traps. A thick mesh is provided at the entry point of the trap to stop the solid particles from entering the trap. The depth of the water seal varies from 50 mm to 75 mm. This trap is not used for collecting soil pipe waste.

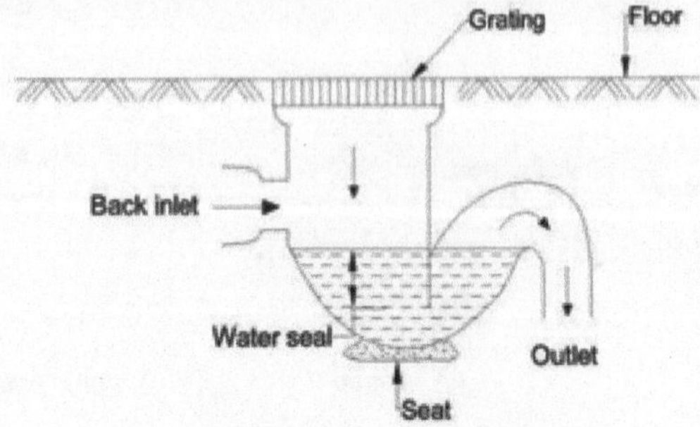

Figure 4.18: Gully trap

c) **Intercepting trap:** These traps are provided at the junction of the domestic sewer from the household and municipal sewer line to prevent the contaminated gases from the municipal sewer to the domestic sewer line from the household as shown in figure 4.20. This type of trap is provided inside a small manhole. The depth of the water seal in this trap is kept from 75 mm to 100 mm. A cleaning eye or loading arm is provided at the top of the trap to clean the trap by inserting a long rod to clean any type of blockage inside the trap. There is a plug provided at the top of the cleaning eye so that contaminated gases do not enter into the building's domestic sewer line by this route. For entering fresh air inside the intercepting chamber the vertical pipes are installed at the top of the chamber. Properly designed interceptors help is easily removal of sewage waste from the building. The installation of interceptor traps affects the ventilation of public sewer which is not favored by engineers. So nowadays the domestic sewer from households is directly connected to the municipal sewer line.

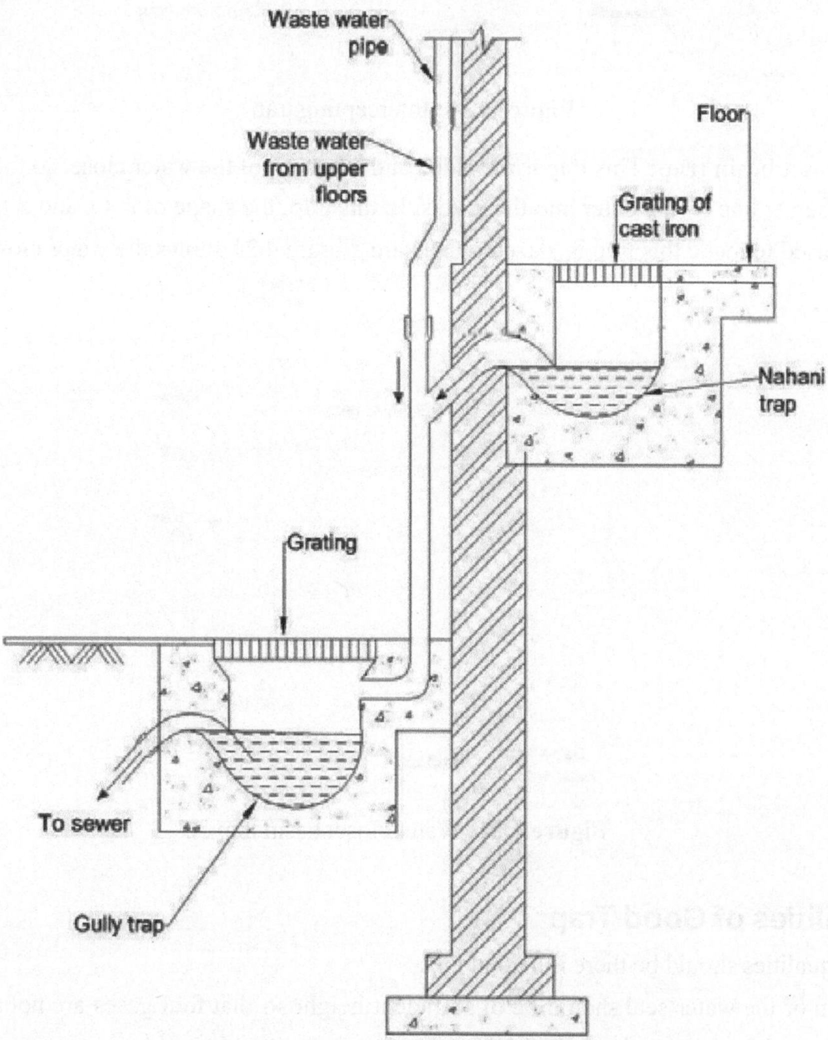

Figure 4.19: Location of floor trap and gully trap

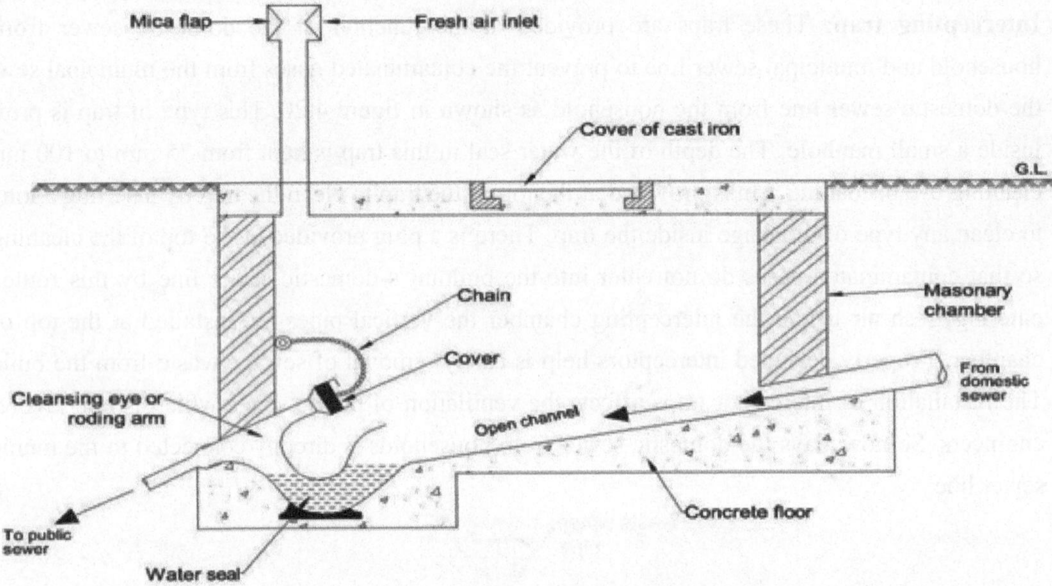

Figure 4.20: Intercepting trap

(d) **Water closet basin trap:** This trap is provided at the bottom of the water closet so that the foul gases from the sewer line do not enter into the toilets. In this trap, the shape of P, Q, and S trap is used. The material used to make this trap is glazed chinaware. Figure 4.21 shows the water closet basin trap.

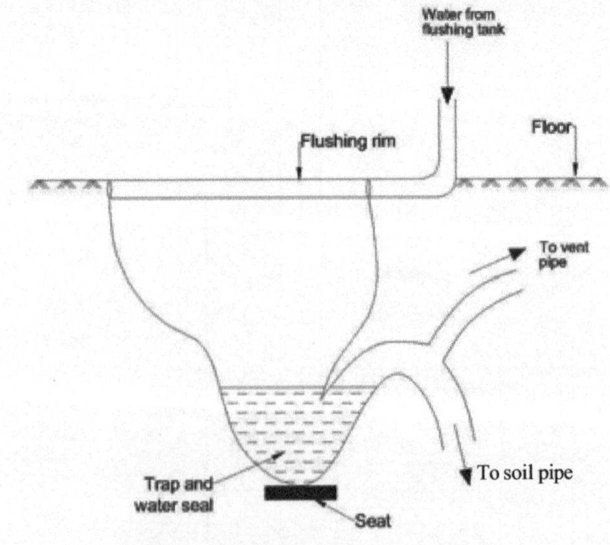

Figure 4.21: Water closet basin trap

4.1.4.1 Qualities of Good Trap

The following qualities should be there is a good trap:

1. The depth of the water seal should be of sufficient height so that foul gases are not able to enter the building if the water exits under high pressure.

2. The inside of the trap should have a smooth surface so that no obstruction occurs to the flowing water.
3. It should be made from water-resistant material so there is no leakage of water from the trap.
4. It should have a simple design and easy to fit.
5. The base of the trap should have a sufficient flat base so that the trap can easily fit
6. In case of blockage of trap it should be easy to clean the blockage of the trap

4.1.6 System of Plumbing

Plumbing involves a water supply pipeline for providing water to the toilets, bathroom, etc., and a drainage pipe for the removal of contaminated water. It involves lying of the pipes. Different systems of plumbing are used to install these fittings. The following systems are explained in below mentioned section.

(1) One pipe plumbing system: In this plumbing system there are two different vertical pipes are fitted. In one vertical pipe, both sewage water and sullage water collect together from different sanitary fittings through different branches and the second vertical pipe is a vent pipe which is used to release the foul gases as shown in figure 4.22. All sanitary fittings from toilets, bathrooms, and sinks on different floors are attached to the vent pipe which helps in maintaining the water seal of the trap. The diameter of the vent pipe is kept at a minimum of 50 mm and the depth of the water seal is maintained at 75 mm. This system is better than the single-stack system. This system is better for multistory buildings.

(2) Two-pipe plumbing system: In this plumbing system there are four different vertical pipes are installed. In these four pipes, there are two sets are made. One set contains the soil pipe and vent pipe for the collection of wastewater from urinals and water closets from different floors. The second set contains a sullage pipe that collects wastewater from the kitchen, sinks, and bathrooms from different floors while the vent pipe present in this set helps in removing the contaminated gas as shown in figure 4.23. A Gully trap is provided at the end of the sullage pipe and in soil pipe there is no need of a gully trap as the drainage pipe is directly connected to the soil pipe. In this system there is amount of pipe used is double that of the one-pipe plumbing system which increases the cost. This system is difficult to fit in a small house as they require a large area to accommodate.

(3) Single stack plumbing system: In this system, there is one pipe that collects waste from toilets, bathrooms, urinals and sinks from different floors. In this system there is no separate vent pipe is provided. In this system sewage and sullage waste are carried through one pipe without ventilation. In this system floor trap is necessary to provide. The cowl is provided at the top of the waste collection pipe. The waste pipe is kept about 2000 mm from the roof to release any harmful gas present in the pipe. Figure 4.24 shows the single-stack system.

4.1.6.1 Choice of system

As discussed in the above article different systems of plumbing, the one-pipe plumbing system is the best method for the effective removal of sewage and sullage waste from toilets, kitchens and bathrooms. This system uses a minimum number of traps and can favor multistory apartments. In this system, the toilets and different sanitary fittings can be fitted at the same place on different floors located above each other. One pipe system can be easy accumulating drainage pipe and is economical in cost. This system can easily be installed in a small house.

4.1.7 Principles regarding the design of building drainage

The principles regarding the design of building drainage are:

i) The soil pipe and sullage pipe waste moved out of the house as soon as possible so that no foul gas can enter the building.

ii) Domestic sewer should be designed in such a way that no overflow occurs during maximum discharge. The domestic sewer should have a pipe with a diameter ranging from 100 to 200 mm.

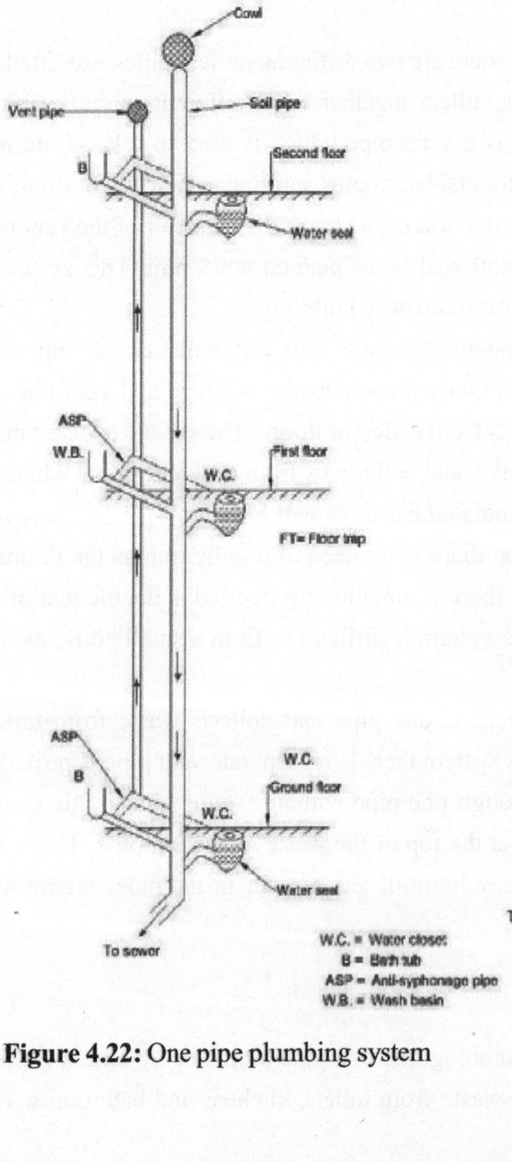

Figure 4.22: One pipe plumbing system

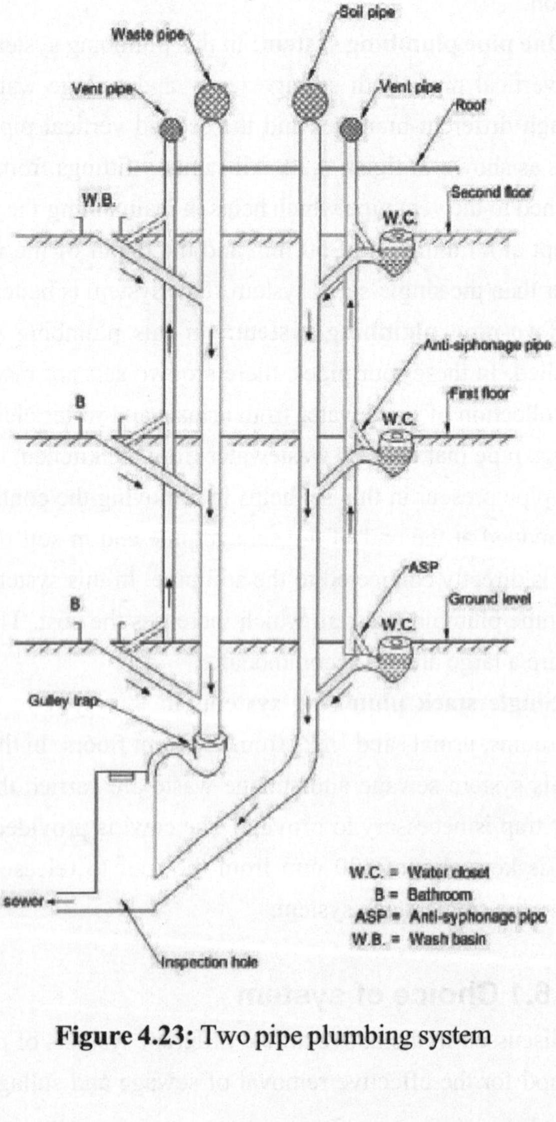

Figure 4.23: Two pipe plumbing system

iii) The velocity inside the drain and domestic pipe should be such that the self-cleaning takes place. For this, the vertical gradient of the pipe should be kept in range from 1in 40 to 1 in 60.

iv) All joints should be waterproof and no leakage from the drain pipes.

v) There should be no right-angle joint of the drain otherwise, they should join by forming a simple curve.

vi) Proper ventilation arrangement made for each drain. The vent pipe should be provided with a drain pipe and this vent pipe should be kept a minimum of 600 mm from the roof.

vii) The overall length of the domestic drain pipe should be kept at a minimum so that inspection can be done easily.

viii) Water seal traps should be provided at the ends of sanitary fittings and proper depth of water seal should be maintained.

4.1.8 Inspection and junction chambers

These chambers are small manholes made for controlling the flow from the domestic sewer, changes in the direction of the flow of domestic sewer, and inspection and cleaning of any blockage in a domestic sewer drain. In these chambers, there is no need for any worker to enter the chamber. They can be inspected by lifting the cover of the chamber by opening the chamber from the top. Blockage can be removed by this chamber using the long rod. This chamber is built up when two or more than two sewer pipes are connected. They are provided when the straight length of the domestic sewer is very long. In that case, they are located at an interval of 10 to 15 m.

They are rectangular and their depth is kept according to the slope of the domestic sewer drain. A rectangular size of 750 mm by 600 mm should be provided for the inspection chamber. The top of the chamber is covered with cast-iron or reinforced cement concrete cover.

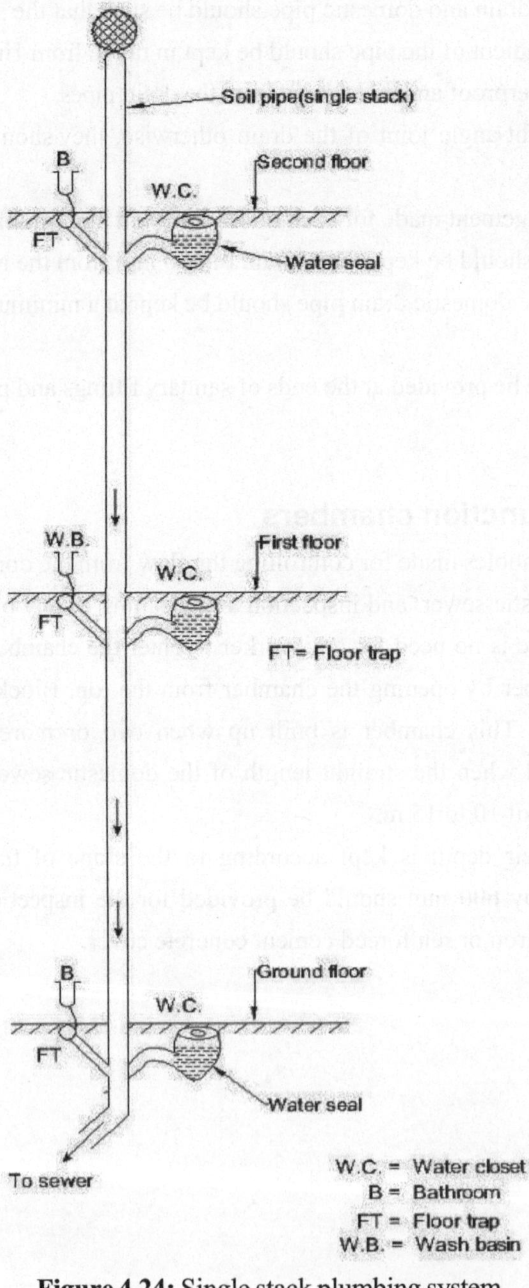

Figure 4.24: Single stack plumbing system

4.2 Systems of Sewerage and Sewer Appurtenances

Sewer pipes are generally laid underground with some slope and they carry sewer water and storm water. These sewer pipes are circular, egg-shaped, semicircular, etc. shape, and sewer water flows under gravitational flow. Some special construction done on sewer lines to control and smooth flowing of sewers is known as sewer appurtenances.

4.2.1 Types of Sewers

Sewers are used to move sewage water out of the town and the type of sewer material used depends on the ease of construction of sewer lines and the cost of construction of pipes. Sewers are classified into different types based on the material used for their construction:

(1) **Glazed stoneware pipe:** This pipe is also known as vitrified clay pipe. This pipe has a diameter ranging from 100 mm to 900 mm and its length varies from 600 mm to 900 mm. It can bear an internal pressure of 1.5 kg/cm^2. The manufacturing of this pipe takes place by heating a special type of soil at 1200°C while heating the pipe a sprinkle of salt is done to make the outer surface shiny and water-proof. This pipe is not affected by corrosion, or acidic, and alkaline sewer water. They are connected by using sockets and spigot joints and are easy to lay. These pipes are mainly used to carry domestic sewer water.

(2) **Cement concrete pipe:** Cement concrete pipes are made for smaller diameters of size less than 450 mm. This pipe is durable and waterproof. Their making is cost-efficient but they are affected by acidic and alkaline sewer water. These pipes are very heavy and difficult to transport as they can easily crack. These pipes are easy to lay and joint. These pipes are made into two types. One is a pressure pipe and the other one is a non-pressure pipe. In a pressure pipe, the sewer flows under pressure while in a non-pressure pipe the sewer flows under gravitational force. Their construction is done as per IS 458-2021.

(3) **Reinforced cement concrete pipe:** A reinforced cement concrete pipe is a concrete pipe that is made by reinforcing steel bars in a circular ring or longitudinal direction so that the pipe can withstand internal and external pressure. These pipes are manufactured in diameters ranging from 600 mm to 1800 mm. Their length is kept at about 1200 mm. This pipe is used when the sewer line has to pass underneath a railway track or main road.

(4) **Hume pipe:** This pipe is a type of reinforced cement concrete pipe in which a steel plate is coated with cement concrete from the inside. The cement coating varies from 12 to 30 mm depending on the diameter of the pipe. This pipe is used to carry sewer when the sewer line passes through the trench. They are waterproof and vibration resistant. They are available in different diameters which vary from 100 mm to 2500 mm. Their length varies from 1000 mm to 3000 mm. They are joined by using a collar joint.

(5) **Cast-iron pipe:** These pipes are stronger pipes that can withstand heavy traffic. This pipe is costlier and they have to protect it from acidic and alkaline sewer water by coating it with bitumen. They are manufactured by sand molding technique and centrifugal process. They are available in diameter varies from 100 mm to 1500 mm. They are made in 2000mm length.

4.2.2 System of sewerage

The following are different systems of sewerage:

(a) **Separate sewerage system:** As the name suggests in this sewerage system there are different sewer lines to carry sewage water and storm water. Figure 4.25 shows the separate sewerage system. This system is used in a town or city where there is very heavy rainfall of more than 750 mm in a year and the rainfall is around 3 to 4 months. This system is easy to lay. As the system is separate the load on the sewage treatment plant is not much as the storm water is directly discharged into the river without treatment. This system is very costly as two separate pipes have to lay. There is one major drawback in this system to maintaining the self-cleaning velocity in the sewer line as there is fluctuation in sewer discharge throughout the day.

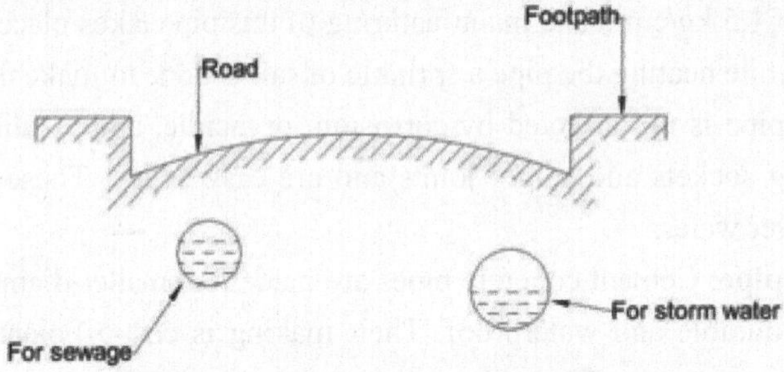

Figure 4.25: Separate sewerage system

(b) **Combined sewerage system:** In this system of sewerage the sewer water and storm water flow in one pipe as seen in figure 4.26. This type of system is very useful in places where the rainfall is less but occurs throughout the year. This system is found in highly dense places where no separate sewer line can be placed due to the limitation of space. This system is easy to maintain and repair as there is only one line for all types of wastewater. This system always has self- cleaning velocity. This system has a larger diameter and is very useful in narrow streets. The main drawback of this system is that in this storm water is also treated before discharge into the river. In this system as having large diameter the excavation is done on a large scale to accumulate larger diameter pipe.

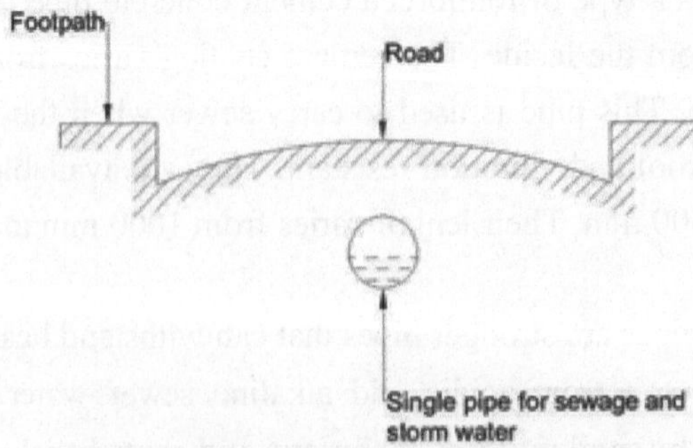

Figure 4.26: Combined sewerage system

(c) **Partially separated sewerage system:** In this system, the rain water from the roof and parking place of the household is discharged into the sewer line while the rainwater from roads and parks is carried by storm drains. This system is a modified type of separate sewerage system. This system works satisfactorily where the rainfall occurs for a few months. This system helps maintain the self-cleaning velocity in the sewer pipe line. Now a days in bigger cities the separated sewerage system is preferred over combined sewerage system. But the separate system cannot be laid in congested part of the city as there is no space to laid two individual pipe and it is costlier to laid two pipes as compared to one. In combined system the sewage water is mixed with storm water and make storm water polluted. Due to which the capacity of treatment plant has to be increased in combined system as compared to separate system. Economic feasibility of the system will depend on the individual town or city project and number of population and size of the town.

4.2.3 Self-cleansing velocity

Self-cleansing velocity is a flow velocity in the sewer pipe that does not allow the suspended matter in sewage to settle down in the pipeline. This velocity is such that it cleans and whips all such suspended matter. Self-cleaning velocity should be maintained once a day so that it automatically cleans all the waste from the sewer pipe. Self-cleansing velocity depends upon the particle size and the specific weight of the particles present in the sewage water. Typically, a minimum of 0.6 m/sec velocity should be maintained in the sewer line to avoid any deposition of suspended matter in the pipeline.

4.2.4 Non-scouring velocity

Non-scouring velocity is the maximum velocity by which sewage water flows in the sewer line without causing any deterioration to the inner surface of the sewer pipe. This velocity depends on the type of materials used for the construction of sewer pipes. Cement concrete pipe is easily worn as compared to glazed stone earthenware pipe. The bottom of the sewer pipeline is more prone to wear as heavy particle flows near the bottom of the pipeline.

4.2.5 Laying of sewers

While during the planning for a town the sewerage system is designed according to the contour plan of the town. Population density and the catchment area the sewer line carries in one sewer line has to be calculated which helps in knowing the diameter of pipe required. In laying the sewer line the pipe is first laid to the outfall end and from there, it is laid inside to the town. This is done so that outfall pipes can be utilized from the start as the pipes are laying and we have not to wait till the completion of the sewerage system.

While laying the pipe first manholes are to be marked on the drawing and then a sewer line is laid between these two manholes. Offset lines are marked on the site and pegs are installed on the offset line at an interval of 15 m and more. From this offset line, the centerline of the sewer drain is marked which is parallel to the offset line, and can be seen in figure 4.27. The excavated soil from the trench should be kept along the excavation side so that it does not disturb the offset points.

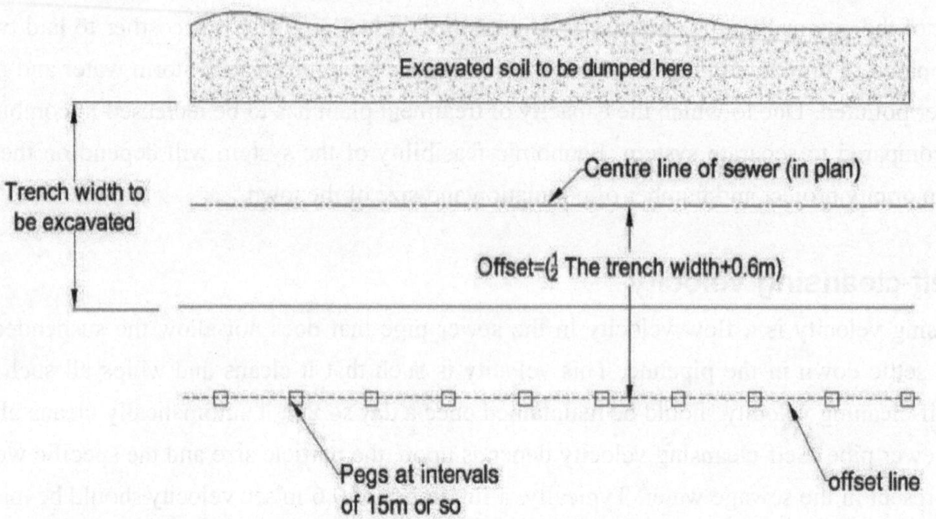

Figure 4.27: Offset line with details

After the centerline is marked the excavation of the trench is done. First, the road pavement is removed from the top surface, and after that hard concrete and soil are removed by using a backhoe to the required depth. The width of the trench is generally 150 mm more than the diameter of the sewer line. For a smaller diameter sewer line, the width is kept a minimum of 600 mm to 750 mm so that laying of pipe and joining of pipe can be done easily. Figure 4.28 shows the excavation of the trench to be done for laying of pipe. If the depth of the trench is more than the wall of the trench is supported by timbering from preventing side soil back into the trench. For smaller depths the wall of the trench is kept vertical. The bottom of the sewer line is made up of plain concrete in which the sewer line is bedded. Smaller diameter pipes are laid down with the help of manpower while the larger diameter pipes are laid using machines. While lowering and joining the sewer line it should be seen that the alignment of the sewer line does not disturb.

4.2.6 Testing and maintenance of sewers

After laying and joining the sewer line they have to be tested for water leakage and their alignments. The tests for checking water leakage and alignment are described in the below section.

1. Test for water leakage: This test is done to ensure that after laying and joining the sewer line there is no water leakage in the sewerage system. In this test the sewer section between two manholes is selected and the water is filled in this selected section with a pressure of 1.5 m water head. While filling the water one end of the sewer line between manholes is covered with a plug and the water is filled with the other end as shown in figure 4.29. After filling the water this sewer pipe line is inspected along the trench line for any water leakage from joints. If there is any leakage found it is repaired or else they replace the joint.

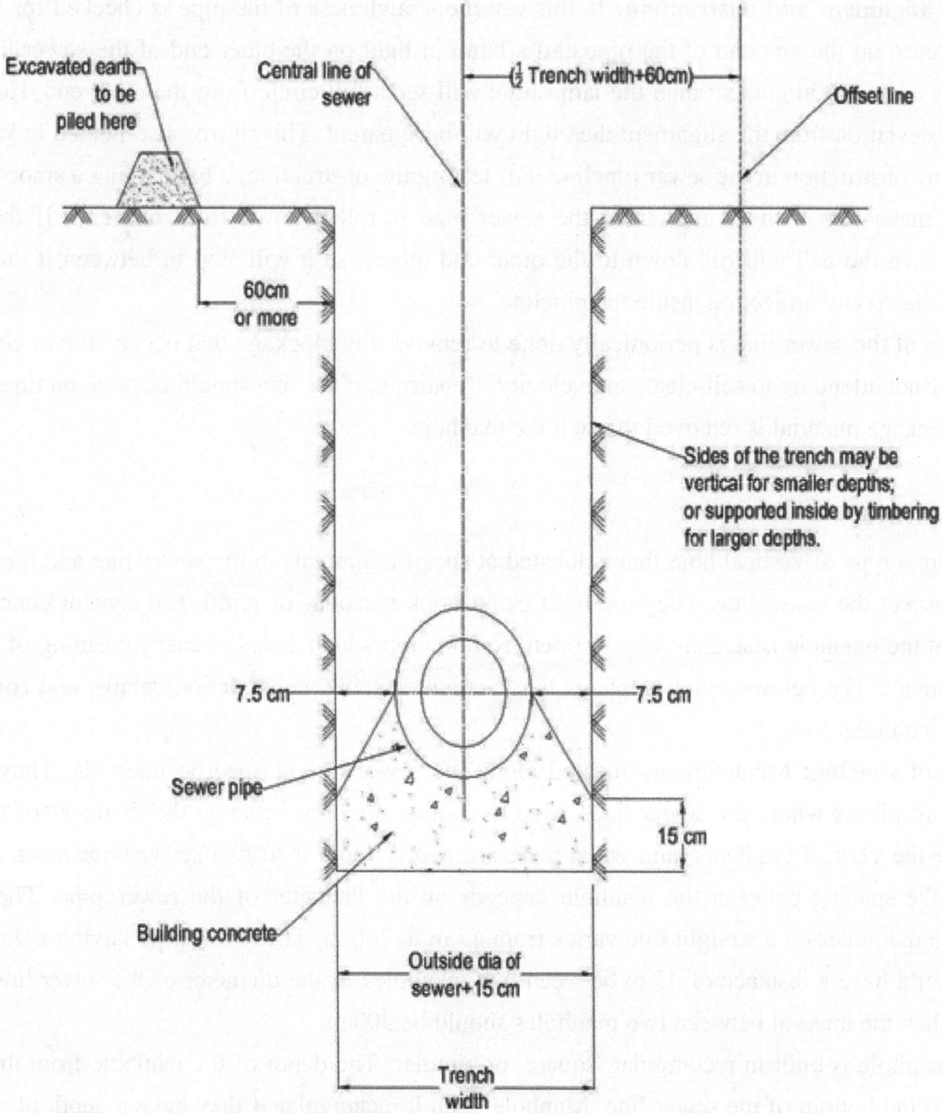

Figure 4.28: Details of excavation of trench

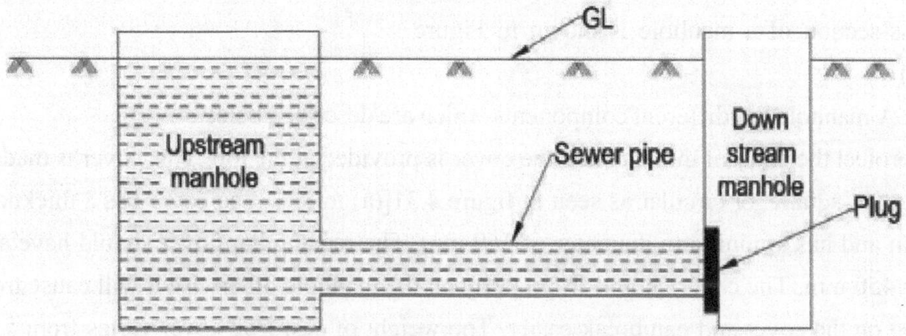

Figure 4.29: Details for water leakage test

2. Test for alignment and obstruction: In this test the straightness of the pipe is checked for which the mirror is placed on the one end of the pipe and a lamp in light on the other end of the sewer line. If the pipeline has a straight alignment then the lamp light will see a full circle from the other end. However, if there is any deviation from the alignment then light will be apparent. This mirror also helped in knowing if there was any obstruction in the sewer pipeline. For testing the obstruction, a ball having a smooth surface and has diameter less than 13 mm from the sewer pipe is rolled down from one end. If there is no obstruction then the ball will roll down to the other end otherwise it will stop in between if there is any obstruction due to any projection inside the pipeline.

Maintenance of the sewer line is periodically done to remove any blockage that occurs due to clogging of the sewer by not attending to self-cleansing velocity. Repairing of the line should be done on time to avoid leakage. Blockage material is removed through the manhole.

4.2.7 Manhole

Manholes are a type of vertical hole that is located at specific intervals in the sewer line and they provide access to inspect the sewer line. They are built using brick masonry or reinforced cement concrete. The sewer line at the manhole is semicircular or open from the top which helps in easily cleaning of sewer by using equipment. The below section explains the location, spacing, construction details, and components parts of the manhole.

Location and spacing: Manholes are located along the sewer line at specific intervals. They are also constructed in places where the sewer lines have to change direction, change the diameter of the sewer line, change the vertical gradients, and when there are two or more than two sewer lines meet. As per IS 1742-1983 the spacing between the manhole depends on the diameter of the sewer pipe. The interval between two manholes on a straight line varies from 45 m to 300 m. The sewer pipe having a diameter of 300 mm should have a distance of 45 m between two manholes. If the diameter of the sewer line is more than 1.5 m then the interval between two manholes should be 300 m.

Shape: A manhole is built in rectangular, square, or circular. The depth of the manhole from the ground level is up to the bottom of the sewer line. Manhole is built rectangular if they have a depth of up to 900 mm from the ground level. When the depth is more than 900 mm the manhole is built in a circular shape. A typical cross-section of a manhole is shown in Figure 4.30 [(a) to (d)].

Components: A manhole has different components which are described below:

i) Cover: To protect the entry of the manhole the cover is provided at the top. This cover is made up of cast iron in rectangular, square, or circular as seen in figure 4.31[(a) to (c)]. The cover has a thickness of about 200 to 250 mm and has a minimum diameter of 560 mm. The rectangular cover should have a dimension of 600 mm by 450 mm. The cover should fit properly on the manhole otherwise it will cause trouble to the vehicle moving on the cover and can break easily. The weight of cast iron cover varies from 51 kg to 255 kg based on traffic moves over the cover. The top surface of the cover has some grooves so that people do not slip while walking over the cover. The groove is made at the edge of the cover and filled with grease so that it fits properly and an airtight joint is formed which helps prevent the escape of contaminated gases.

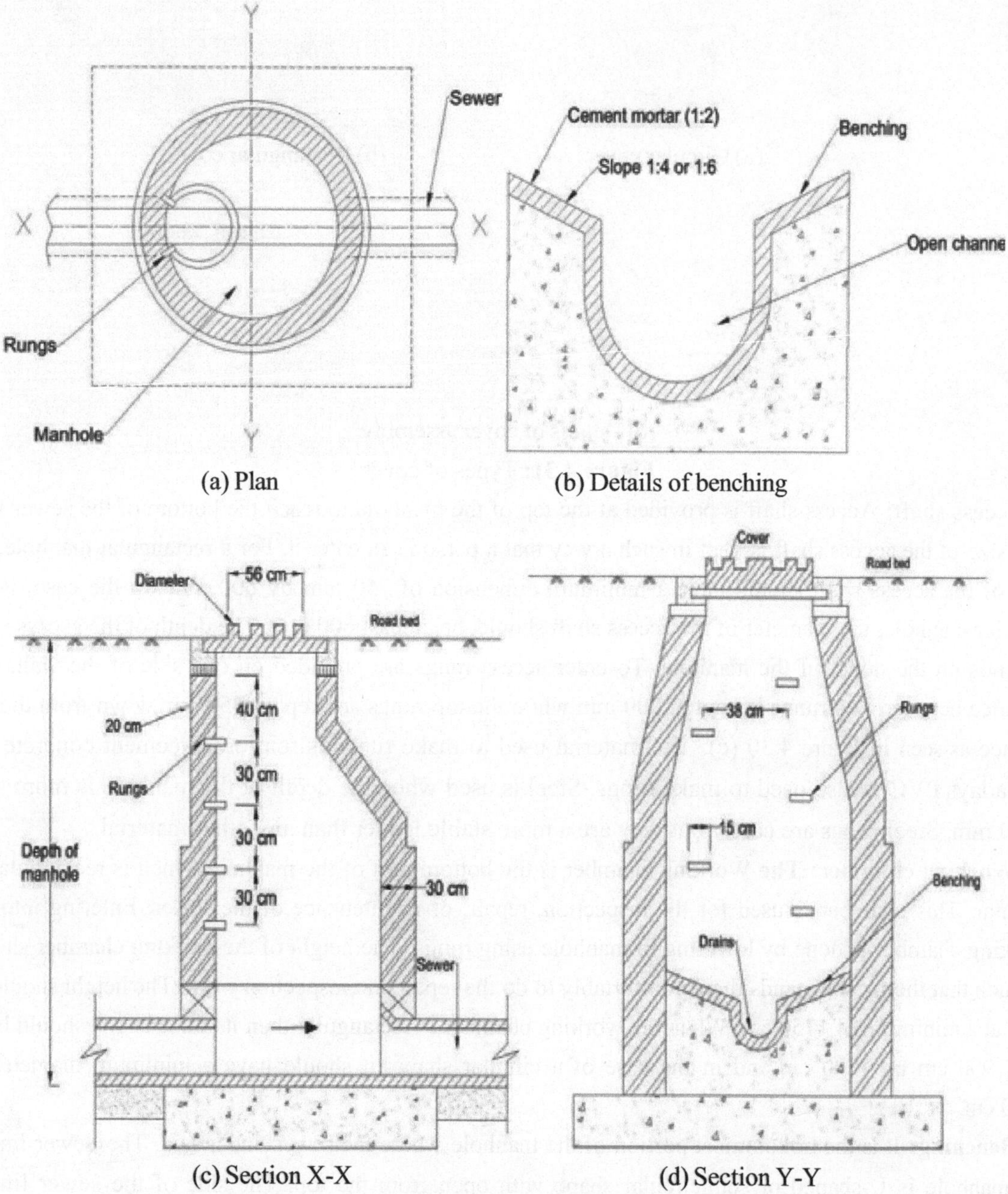

Figure 4.30: Manhole

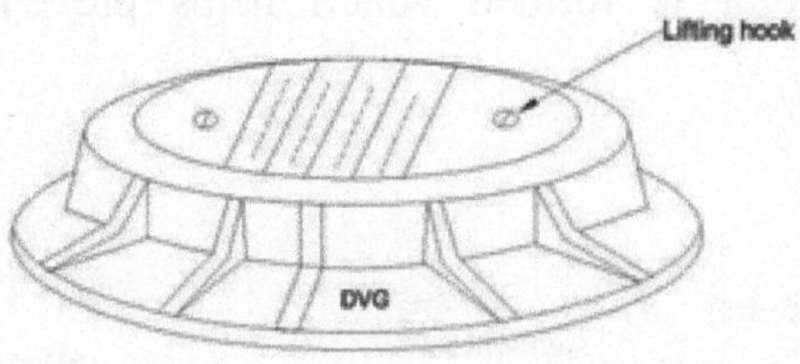

(a) Circular cover

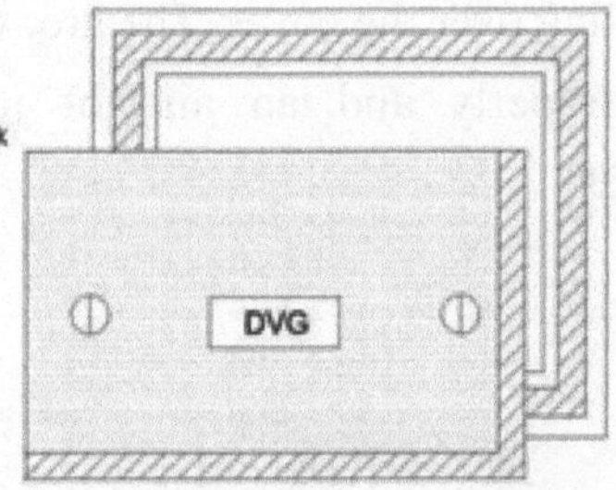

(b) Rectangular cover

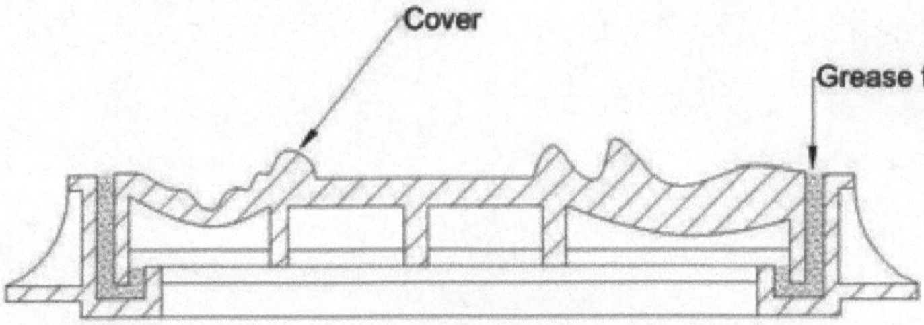

(c) Details of cover assembly

Figure 4.31: Types of cover

ii) Access-shaft: Access-shaft is provided at the top of the manhole to reach the bottom of the sewer line. The size of the access shaft is kept in such a way that a person can enter it. For a rectangular manhole, the size of the access shaft should have a minimum dimension of 750 mm by 600 mm. In the case of the circular manhole, the diameter of the access shaft should be at least 600 mm. The depth of the access shaft depends on the depth of the manhole. To enter access rungs are provided on one side of the wall. The distance between two rungs is kept at 300 mm while the top rungs are kept at 450 mm down from the top surface as seen in figure 4.30 (c). The material used to make rungs is reinforced cement concrete but nowadays PVC is also used to make rungs. Steel is used when the depth of the manhole is more than 6000 mm. Steel rungs are costly but they are a more stable ladder than any other material.

iii) Working chamber: The Working chamber is the bottom part of the manhole which is rectangular or circular. This chamber is used for the inspection, repair, or maintenance of the sewer. Entering into the working chamber is done by lowering in manhole using rungs. The height of the working chamber should be such that the person stands there comfortably to do the repair and inspection work. The height should be kept at a minimum of 1750 cm. When the working chamber is rectangular then its dimensions should be at least 900 cm by 1200 cm and in the case of a circular shape, it should have a minimum diameter of 1200 cm.

iv) Benching: It is the bottommost portion of the manhole where the sewer line is laid. The sewer line in the manhole is U-shaped or semicircular shape with open from the top. The side of the sewer line is somewhat slope which varies from 1:4 to 1:6 as shown in figure 4.30 (b). The concreting done on the top of the sewer line to make the slope is known as benching.

Construction details: The exact location of the manhole is decided before installing the sewer line. Excavation of soil is done for laying the manhole. The foundation of the manhole is done by cement concrete. The thickness of cement concrete at the base of the foundation varies from 150 mm to 250 mm depending on the depth of the manhole. Brick masonry, stone masonry, or concrete is used to build the sides of manholes. Plastering is done on side walls from inside and outside using cement mortar (1:5). There is a thumb rule given to calculate the thickness of the side wall.

$$T=10+4d$$

Where T = Side wall thickness in cm d = excavation depth in m

When reinforced cement concrete is used to build a side wall then the thickness is calculated by structural analysis methods and it is less than the brick masonry.

4.2.8 Drop Manhole

Drop manhole is constructed in places where the main sewer line and branches sewer line are not is the same plan but have a vertical difference of around 600 mm at the intersection.

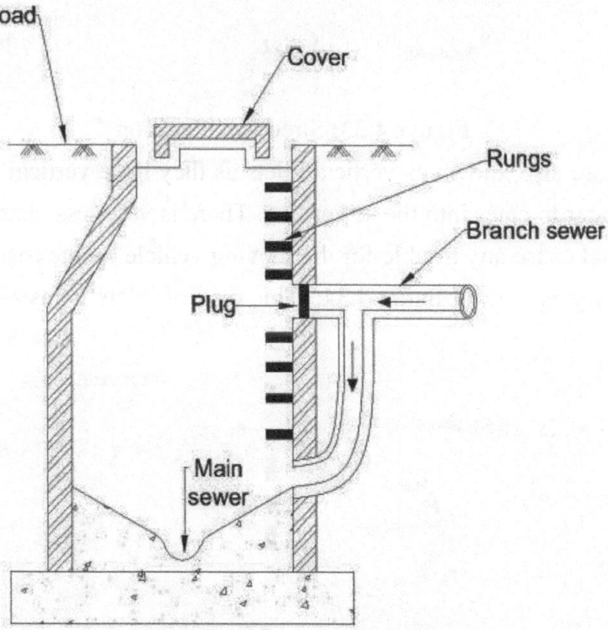

Figure 4.32: Drop manhole

In this branch sewer line is joined to main sewer line with the help of a vertical pipe as shown in figure 4.32. A plug is inserted into the end of the branch sewer line at the intersection on the manhole side wall. Scan code is given for extra information about drop manhole.

4.2.9 Street inlets and sewer inlets

Street inlets are used to collect road surface water. They are made at an interval of 30 m to 60 m on the straight road on both sides. They are also located at each corner of the intersection of the road as shown in figure 4.33. Thick cast iron mesh is provided at the mouth of these inlets to stop the entry of organic matter such as large tree branches, paper, falling leaves, etc. This also helps in preventing the entry of animals. These inlets are connected to the main sewer line by making a manhole at the center of the road. The pipes used to carry the street inlets to the sewer line should have a minimum diameter of 200 mm. The street inlets are joined to the sewer line by the help of traps so that the water seal is maintained and contaminated gases from the sewer line do not come out from the street inlets. These street inlets are made up of cement concrete or brick masonry. They are of two types depending on the opening of the inlet.

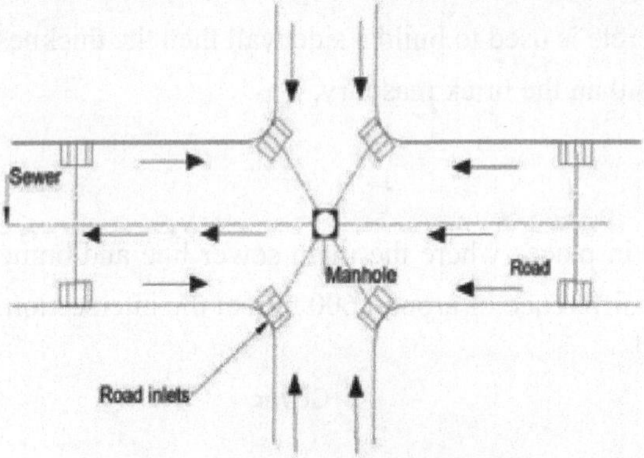

Figure 4.33: Street inlet location

i. **Kerb inlet:** They are also known as vertical inlets as they have vertical opening on the side of the footpath for rainwater to enter into the sewer line. There is very less chance of the blockage of kerb inlet and they do not cause any trouble for the moving vehicle on the road as there opening is inside the footpath masonry as seen in figure 4.34. This type of inlets is installed on roads having heavy traffic movement.

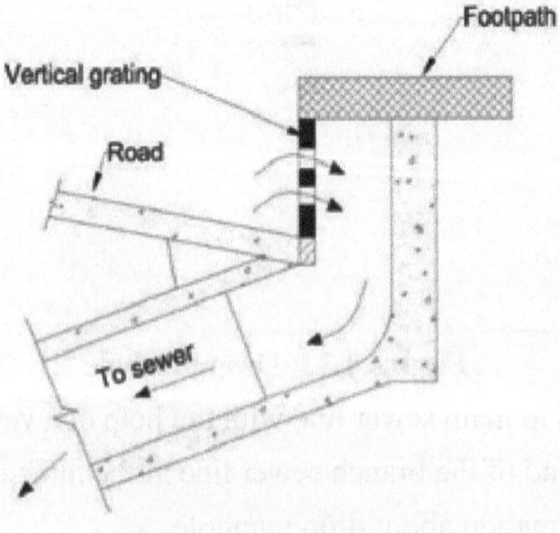

Figure 4.34: Kerb inlet

ii. **Gutter inlet:** They are also known as horizontal inlets as they have horizontal opening over the drain on the side of road. The side of the road has a slope such that all the rainwater from road reaches to the inlets. In this inlets large amount of water moves rapidly but there is draw back in this inlets as there is a chance that heavy vehicle can break the inlets as they are very heavy. Figure 4.35 shows the gutter inlets.

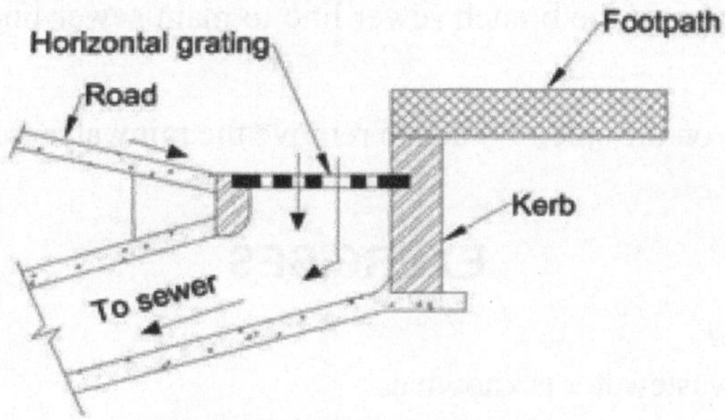

Figure 4.35: Gutter inlet

UNIT SUMMARY

- Different technical terms related to building sanitation are explained
- Various building sanitation fittings such as water closet, Flushing cistern, wash basin, etc are explained
- Sewage pipe is used to carry toilet sewage and sullage pipe carries waste from kitchen and sinks.
- Indian water closet and European water closet are discussed in detail
- Flushing cistern design details are explained and its types are discussed
- Flat back and pedestal wash basin are discussed in detail
- Different types of urinals as per their uses are explained.
- Traps are provided at the bottom of building sanitary fittings to prevent enter of contaminated gases in the house.
- P-traps and S-traps are generally used in sanitary fittings.
- Traps classification based on uses are discussed
- Various qualities of traps are discussed to select the perfect trap as per their uses.
- Plumbing system is described which involves fittings of pipes
- One pipe plumbing systems are best suited for multi-story buildings.
- Principles regarding the design of building drainage are discussed.
- Different types of sewer pipes are explained
- Separate sewerage system is most useful for places having heavy rainfall for 3 to 4 months in a year
- A partially separated sewerage system is the most economical of all the other types of sewerage system.
- Sewer pipes should be designed in such a way that self-cleansing velocity should always maintained.
- How the sewer lines laid in the underground soil is explained
- Test for the water leakage and alignments are discussed for sewer line
- Manhole is providing at the junction of sewer line to inspect the sewer line and for repair and maintenance.

- Drop manhole is used to join the branch sewer line to main sewer line when both line have vertical difference.
- Street inlets are provide on the side of roads to remove the rainwater from the streets

EXERCISES

Multiple Choice Questions

1. Bathroom and kitchen wastewater is known as
   (a) Sullage waste (b) Sewage waste
   (c) Refuse waste (d) none of the above
2. What is the minimum diameter used for rainwater pipe?
   (a) 200 mm (b) 150 mm
   (c) 250 mm (d) 175 mm
3. Which pipe is used to remove contaminated gases from the toilet?
   (a) Sewage pipe (b) Soil pipe
   (c) Vent pipe (d) All of the above
4. Bell-type flushing cistern is a type of……..
   (a) Valve less symphonic action (b) valve symphonic action
   (c) Tube symphonic action (d) None
5. Bowl-type urinal has a flushing cistern installed at a minimum height of…..
   (a) 2000 mm (b) 1900 mm
   (c) 2500 mm (d) 2200 mm
6. Traps based on shapes are classified as
   (a) P-trap (b) S-trap
   (c) Q-trap (d) Y-trap
7. Which system of sewerage collects both sewer waste and storm sewer together
   (a) Separate sewerage system (b) Combined sewerage system
   (c) Partially separated sewerage system (d) None of the above
8. Which pipe is used to protect the water seal of the traps?
   (a) Anti-siphonage pipe (b) Sullage pipe
   (c) Sewage pipe (d) None
9. Which test is used to check the leakage in the sewage pipe
   (a) Water test (b) Air test
   (c) Temperature test (d) All of the above
10. Vertical opening is provided in which type of street inlets
    (a) Kerb inlet (b) Gutter inlets
    (c) Storm inlets (d) All of the above
11. What is the minimum diameter used for rainwater pipe?
    (a) 120 mm (b) 100 mm
    (c) 150 mm (d) None

Answers to Multiple Choice Questions

1. (a), 2. (b), 3. (c), 4. (a), 5. (b), 6. (d), 7. (b), 8. (a), 9. (a) 10. (a) 11. (b)

Short and Long Answer Type Questions

1. Explain the difference between sewage waste and sullage waste.
2. Write a short note on Rainwater pipe and vent pipe.
3. Why are traps installed in building sanitary fittings? Explain briefly.
4. What are the qualities of good traps?
5. Explain the floor trap with a neat diagram.
6. Explain different types of plumbing systems. Which system is more commonly used?
7. Draw a neat diagram of the Indian water closet and explain the position of the traps.
8. Write a short note on the flushing cistern.
9. Explain different types of wash basins with neat diagram.
10. Why and where inspection chamber installed in the building sanitation.
11. Draw a neat diagram of a pipe plumbing system. Explains various components.
12. What are the different tests conducted on sewage pipelines?
13. What are the principles regarding the design of building drainage.
14. Difference between separate sewerage system and combined sewerage system.
15. What are the different types of sewer based on the material used for the construction of sewer pipes?
16. Explain self-cleansing velocity and non-scouring velocity.
17. Write a short note on the lying of sewers.
18. Write a short note on street inlets.
19. Draw a neat sketch of the manhole. Identify its various components.
20. Explain the drop manhole with a diagram.

REFERENCES AND SUGGESTED READINGS

1. Sharma S.C, Environmental Engineering, Khanna Publishing House, New Delhi
2. Garg, S.K., Environmental Engineering Vol. I and Vol. II, Khanna Publishers
3. Birdie, G. S. and Birdie, J. S. Water Supply and Sanitary Engineering, Dhanpat Rai
4. Gupta, O.P., Elements of Environmental Pollution Control, Khanna Publishing House, Delhi
5. Rao, C.S., Environmental Pollution Control Engineering, New Age International
6. Punmia, B C, Environmental Engineering, vol. I and II, Laxmi Publishers
7. Peavy H S, Rowe D R, and Tchobanoglous G, Environmental Engineering, McGraw
8. Basak N N, Environmental Engineering, McGraw Hill Publishers.
9. IS 774-2004, IS 771-1979, IS 2556(part 6)-2021, IS 458-2021 and IS 1742-1983

5 Characteristics and Treatment of Sewage

UNIT SPECIFICS

Through this unit we have discussed the following aspects:

- *To understand the characteristics of sewage and its significance*
- *Different discharge norms for sewage effluent*
- *Overview of screening and grit chamber*
- *Overview of aerobic and anaerobic treatment unit*
- *Discussion on the sludge digestion process*
- *Introduction of septic tank*

The figures are provided in 2D to help the students visualize the content and enhance their practical knowledge. The content in this unit provides practical knowledge that will help the students make decisions during the fieldwork.

This unit contains short and long answer-type questions along with multiple choice questions, a list of references, and suggested reading is given so that one can go through them for practice. Some QR codes are given which can be scanned for more information on various topics of interest and to get extra knowledge.

RATIONALE

This unit on the characteristics and treatment of sewage helps the students to develop an idea about the characteristics of sewage. It explains the process of the treatment of sewage. The various treatment units used for sewage treatment are discussed. A brief discussion of the physical, chemical, and biological characteristics are explained. The various types of screening are also discussed and a grit chamber and skimming tank is given. The content covered in this unit is important to understand which treatment is used for particular characteristics.

The knowledge of analysis and treatment of sewage is essential for civil engineering students. The students can apply the knowledge of the sewage treatment plant construction during their fieldwork. The knowledge gained in this unit will help the students to identify suitable treatment units for different field conditions. The students can apply their knowledge in the selection and implementation of disposal of sewage methods during the sludge disposal. The concepts in this unit will help the student in effective supervision of sewage treatment plants for domestic wastewater.

PRE-REQUISITES

A basic knowledge of water is required.

UNIT OUTCOMES

The list of outcomes of this unit is as follows:

U5-O1: *To explain the process to analyzing the characteristics of sewage.*

U5-O2: *To understand different norms for the discharge of sewage.*

U5-O3: *To realize the suitability of different treatment units for the different sewage characteristics.*

U5-O4: *To determine the function and suitability of aerobic and anaerobic treatment process.*

U5-O5: *To propose a suitable sewage treatment plant.*

Unit-5 Outcomes	EXPECTED MAPPING WITH COURSE OUTCOMES (1- Weak Correlation; 2- Medium correlation; 3- Strong Correlation)				
	CO-1	CO-2	CO-3	CO-4	CO-5
U5-O1	1	-	1	1	3
U5-O2	-	-	1	-	2
U5-O3	1	1	-	-	3
U5-O4	2	1	-	-	3
U5-O5	-	-	-	-	3

5.1 Analysis of sewage

Sewage wastewater and sullage wastewater collected from toilets, kitchens, sinks, bathrooms, hospitals, commercial buildings, etc. must be treated before the water is disposed into the river. As this waste contains organic matter, suspended particles, etc. so, it is necessary to know the concentration in sewage as it will decide the type of treatment required for particular waste before disposal. If proper treatment is not given it will contaminate the river with harmful bacteria. The knowledge of the quality and characteristics of the sewage helps in deciding the disposal method used for a particular type of sewage. Therefore in this chapter, we will discuss the various characteristics of sewage, their treatment and disposal methods.

5.1.1 Characteristics of sewage

The quality if sewage can be checked by analyzing, its physiochemical biological characteristics, as mentioned below.

5.1.1.1 Physical characteristics

To know the physical characteristics of sewage following tests are required on the sewage wastewater.

i. **Turbidity:** Sewage wastewater is highly turbid water that contains waste from toilets, bathrooms, and kitchens. Sewage wastewater turbidity increases as the sewage strength increases. The turbidity of sewage is calculated in the same manner as calculated in Chapter 1, "Sources, demand and Quality of Water".

ii. **Colour:** The color of the sewage wastewater can be seen through the naked eye. If the color of sewage waste water is grey or yellowish it indicates the sewage is fresh while if the color is dark brown or black it indicates the sewage is older and stale. Sometimes the color of the sewage can be different than the above-mentioned color due to the presence of specific waste from the industries.

iii. **Odour:** Fresh wastewater does not foul smell it is an odor but as time passes it starts to give a foul and rotten smell. This smell occurs when all the oxygen gas present in the wastewater is consumed. Hydrogen sulfide gas starts to get released as the decomposition of sewage takes place. The threshold odor number is used to measure the odor of the sewage. In this, the sewage sample is diluted using an odorless solution till the sewage becomes odor-free. The minimum odorless solution used to make sewage odor-free is known as the threshold odor number of the sewage.

iv. **Temperature:** Temperature plays a very important role in the decomposition of the organic and inorganic matter present in the sewage as all the biological activity that occurs in the sewage is affected by the increase or decrease of the temperature. Temperature variation also affects the solubility of different gases in sewage. The temperature of sewage water is generally higher than the supplied water. In India, the average temperature of sewage is around 20°C. This average temperature is very ideal for the occurrence of biological activities in sewage.

5.1.1.2 Chemical characteristics

To know the chemical characteristics of sewage following tests are required on the sewage wastewater. This parameter helps in deciding the type of treatment useful for the complete degradation of organic and inorganic matter and the extent of the treatment for making the sewage safe for disposal in rivers.

i. **Solids:** The amount of the solids present are sewage is much less as compared to the amount of water. The amount of solids varies from 0.05% to 0.10% of total sewage. Different forms in which solids present in sewage are suspended, dissolved, settled, and colloidal. Suspended solids remain floating in sewage while dissolved solids dissolve in sewage. Settled solids are heavy solid that settles at the bottom of the tank if remain still for more than 2 hours. Colloidal solids are very small fine particles.

The quality of solids in 1000 kg of sewage is approximately 450 gm, out of which suspended solid is 225 gm, dissolved solid is 112 gm and settable solid is 112 gm. The solids can also be categorized based on their organic and inorganic content. About 55% of the total solid consists of inorganic matter and 45% consists of organic matter. The waste contains nitrogenous compounds, fats, oil, animal waste, etc. are comes under organic waste while inorganic waste contains sand, silts gravels, etc.

Total solids in sewage can be calculated by evaporating the known volume of sewage sample in a crucible and weighing the residual left on the crucible. The total solid will be represented by the weight on the crucible divided by the known volume of the sample taken. Its unit is mg/l or PPM.

Suspended solids can be measured by filtering the known amount of sewage sample through micro filter paper (pore size 1μm). In this the amount which residue on the filter paper is weighed and divided by the known amount of sample used for filtration. Its unit is mg/l or PPM. The difference between the total solid and suspended solids gives the dissolved solid plus colloidal solids. Settable solids are calculated with the help of the instrument Imhoff cone. Imhoff cone is made up of glass that has a conical shape and a capacity is 1 liter and it is graduated from the bottom to the top side and has 10 ml to 50 ml marks as seen in figure 5.1. In the Imhoff cone, the sewage sample is allowed to settle for 2 hours and the amount of solids that settle at the bottom of the cone can be read directly through graduated readings.

ii. pH: The pH of the sewage sample is calculated in the same a way as done for the water sample and explained in Chapter 1 "Sources, demand and Quality of Water". The pH of fresh sewage water is somewhat alkaline i.e. it has pH higher than 7 but as time passes the decomposition of sewage takes place which acidic gas is generated which turns the pH to acidic. pH of sewage is calculated in the same manner as calculated in Chapter 1, "Sources, demand and quality of water".

iii. Chloride content: Chloride content in the domestic sewage comes from kitchen waste and toilet waste. The permissible limit of chloride in water is 250 mg/l and for domestic sewage it is 120 mg/l. However the industrial waste from different industries having chloride increases the chloride content of the domestic sewage. If there is any increase of chloride in the domestic sewage it indicates that industrial waste is discharging in domestic sewage or seawater intrusion is taking place. The testing of chloride in domestic sewage is done by titrating the sewage with silver nitrate solution, an indicator used in this test is potassium chromate.

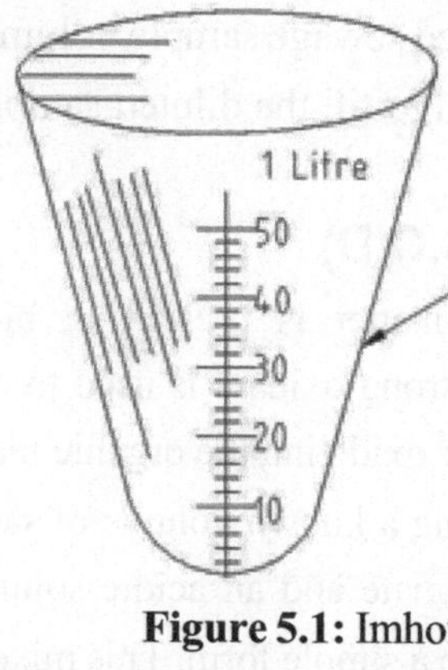

Figure 5.1: Imhoff cone

iv. Presence of Fats, oils, and Greases: Fats, grease, and oils come in the domestic sewage from kitchen waste from households, restaurants, and hotels. The scum formation takes place on the top surface of the sedimentation tanks due to this sewage. This type of waste also clogs the filter media. Special focus has to be given during treatment of such domestic waste. The amount of fats and grease in the sewage is calculated by using the knowledge that these compounds are dissolved in ether. So we mix the fat and grease in the ether solution and evaporated the ether and measure the amount of residue left in the beaker. This left residual give the amount of fat and grease in sewage.

5.1.2 Bio-chemical Oxygen Demand (B.O.D)

B.O.D. of sewage gives the amount of oxygen required by biologically active bacteria to decompose or degrade the organic matter present in a specific period. BOD test in most important test in domestic sewage as it give the proportion of organic matter in sewage. The units used to measure the demand are mg/l.

The BOD is calculated using the standard temperature of 20°C and the duration is 5 days. The demand given by the 5-day test is known as standard demand and about 70% decomposition of total organic matter takes place. If the duration is kept for 10 days then about 90% of organic matter is decomposed of total organic matter. The amount of BOD helps in deciding the strength of the sewage. If the BOD of sewage for 5 days is around 250 mg/l then this type of sewage is known as weak sewage. If this valve is more than 450 mg/l then this type of sewage is known as strong sewage. It means it has a quantity of organic matter.

BOD test in the laboratory is done by dilution method. In this test, the known volume of sewage sample is diluted using distilled water and this sample is kept at 20°C in a biological incubator for 5 days. The dissolved oxygen of the sample before placing it in biological incubation is recorded. After 5 days the dissolved oxygen of the sample is again measured. The difference between the initial dissolved oxygen and after 5 days of dissolved oxygen will give the amount of oxygen consumed by bacteria to decompose the organic matter. The BOD is calculated by using equation 5.1.

$$5\ day\ BOD = Dissolved\ oxygen\ consumed\ in\ 5\ days\ X \frac{\boldsymbol{diluted\ sample\ volume}}{\boldsymbol{undiluted\ sewage\ sample\ volume}} \quad 5.1$$

The ratio of diluted sample volume to undiluted sewage sample volume is known as the dilution factor. In the laboratory, a 300 ml glass bottle is used to fill the diluted sample and incubate it for 5 days.

5.1.3 Chemical Oxygen Demand (C.O.D)

COD is the method in which the organic matter is present in biodegradable as well as in non-biodegradable form in sewage. In this test, a strong oxidant is used to oxidize the sewage organic matter and to determine the amount of oxygen used for oxidizing the organic matter.

In the laboratory, this test is performed by taking a known volume of sample in a borosilicate glass vessel and this sample is mixed with potassium chromate and an acidic solution of H_2SO_4. This strong acid is used to digest and break the complex matter into a simple form. This mixer is placed on a COD digester at a temperature of 150°C for 2 hours. Potassium chromate in the presence of strong acid helps in the digestion of organic matter. The glass vessel is left to cool down at room temperature and after that, the sample is titrated with ferrous ammonium sulfate and ferroin is used as an indicator which gives the amount of oxygen consumed to oxidize the sewage sample. This method is known as the closed reflux method.

5.1.4 Central Pollution Control Board norms for discharge of treated sewage

Central Pollution Control Board norms for discharge for treated sewage as per the Environmental (Protection) Act, 1986 (2016), Ministry of Environment, Forest and Climate Change are as follows:

i) It mentions that in case the sewage after treatment has to be disposed into the sea, then the discharge should have been 100 meters from the shore and should have a minimum of 1500 times dilution. Then the existing norms of general discharge should be followed which is given in table 5.1.

ii) More use of reused/recycled treated sewage be encouraged and in case the reused water comes in contact with humans then existing norms of general discharge should be followed.

iii) All units in table 5.1 are in mg/l except for pH

iv) The general discharge norms are valid for the disposal of treated sewage into water bodies and lands.

General standards for the discharge of environmental pollutants for effluent are given in Schedule VI, Environmental (Protection) Act, 1986 (2016) which is mentioned in below section in Table 5.1

Table 5.1: Permissible limit of effluents as per standard

S. no.	Parameters	Standards		
		Inland Surface water	**Public sewers**	**Land for irrigation**
1	pH	5.5 – 9.0	5.5 – 9.0	5.5 – 9.0
2	Suspended solids	100	600	200
3	Oil and grease	10	20	10
4	BOD (for 3 days at 27°C)	30	350	100
5	COD	250	-	-
6	Ammonical nitrogen	50	50	-
7	Free Ammonia	5.0	-	-
8	Total Kjeldahi nitrogen	100	-	-
9	Arsenic	0.2	0.2	0.2
10	Lead	0.1	0.1	-
11	Cadmium	2.0	1.0	-

A few effluent standards are mentioned in table 5.1. Complete details for all parameters and different industries' effluent can be seen by scanning the QR code given here using mobile. This complete list of parameter and their discharge limit is very important for students to design sewage treatment plants.

5.1.5 Objectives of sewage treatment plant

The main objectives of sewage treatment plants are as follows:

i) Sewage treatment plants help in reducing the organic load which in turn reduces the strength of the sewage and makes it suitable to discharge into the river without polluting river water.

ii) To make the effluent fit for irrigation purpose.

iii) To reduce the strength of sewage solids for safe disposal on land

iv) It should remove the harmful pathogenic bacteria to a level for safely disposed for sewage without effecting human health

5.1.6 Flow diagram of conventional sewage treatment plant

Figure 5.2 shows the flow diagram of conventional sewage treatment

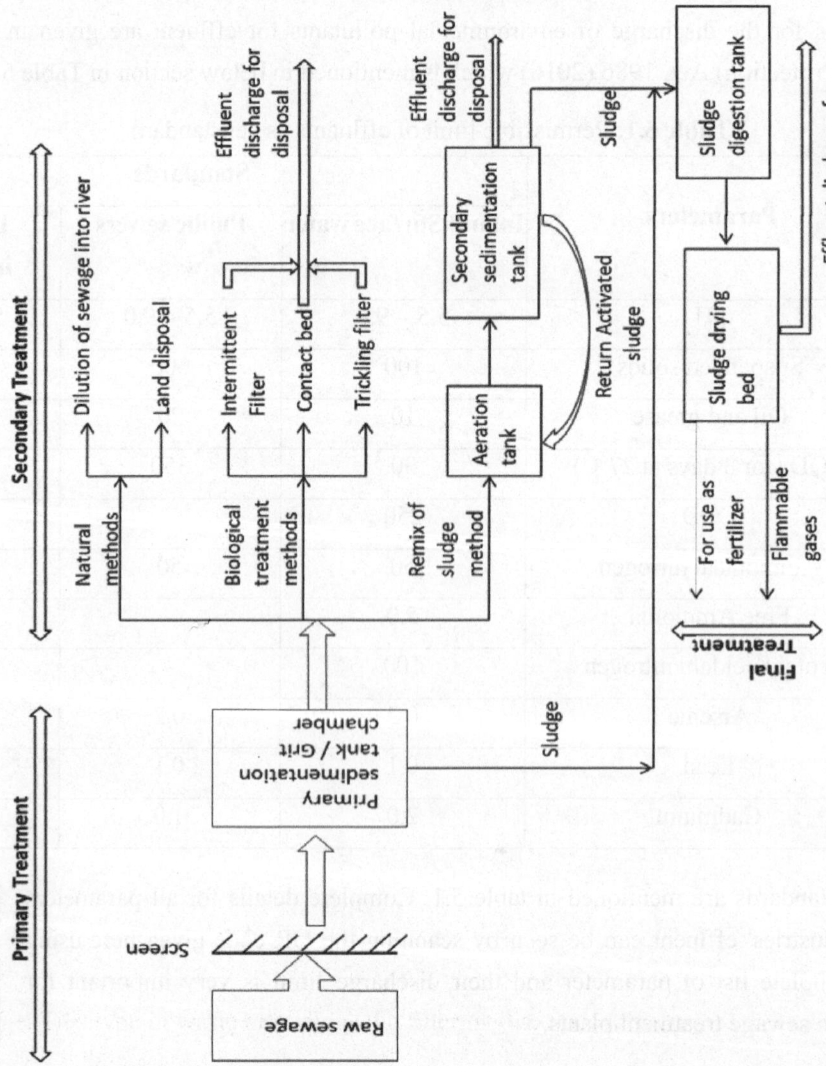

Figure 5.2: Flow diagram of conventional sewage treatment plant

5.2 Treatment of sewage

Treatment of sewage depends on the characteristics of sewage which have been discussed in the analysis of sewage section. Different treatment stages depend on the organic and inorganic content of sewage. These stages are generally classified into 3 stages which can be seen in figure 5.2. The name of treatment stages are:

1. Primary treatment
2. Secondary treatment
3. Final treatment

In primary treatment the suspended impurities which are floating in sewage are removed. Heavy inorganic impurities are also separated from sewage and settled at the bottom in the form of primary sludge. In this process around 30 % of BOD removed from sewage. In this process following treatment unit includes screening, grit chamber, skimming tank and primary sedimentation tank.

In secondary treatment, the sewage effluent from the primary sedimentation tank is further treated to remove dissolved impurities. In this process, biological action takes place to remove or kill pathogenic bacteria and reduce organic load. Aerobic and anaerobic bacteria are used for the decomposition of organic matter. In this treatment BOD is removed up to 90%. Various biological treatment processes are there and can be used according to the characteristics of sewage and to achieve the desired safe limit of effluent to discharge into rivers or seas.

In the final treatment, the sludge from the primary and secondary sedimentation tanks and other treatment units is further processed. The sludge is digested using a sludge digester to decompose waste sludge. After sludge digestion, the harmful bacteria is completely removed and this sludge can be used for farming.

The various combinations of treatment units from primary, secondary, and final treatment are arranged as per the degree of treatment required for sewage treatment before disposal into rivers or land. Various treatment units are discussed in the below-mentioned sections.

5.2.1 Screening

This is the very first treatment operation carried out in the sewage treatment plants. In this process the sewage is passed thought various sizes of screens placed at the inlet of the sewage treatment plant. The floating waste such as cloth, leaves, wood, large plastics, etc. is removed from the sewage with the help of screens. If we do not remove these floating suspended materials they will choke the pipes lines and pumps of the treatment plants. Screens used for removing floating particles are made up of thick wire or metal rods. These screens can be static or mechanically operated.

5.2.2 Types of screening

Screening based on the opening of the mesh or holes is classified into the following types:

i) Coarse screen
ii) Medium screen
iii) Fine screen

In a sewage treatment plant, these screens are arranged in sequences as the first screen is the coarse screen then the medium and at last the fine screen. A detailed explanation of types of careen is explained in the below section.

i) Coarse screen: Coarse screens are placed at the starting inlet point of sewage in the treatment plant. They are used to separate the larger size impurities from the sewage. The size of the opening of the mesh is kept more than 50 mm. The screen has thick mesh or rod arranged to make a small square-shaped opening. These mesh or rods are arranged vertically or diagonally at an angle between 30º to 60º. The screen which is at an angle to the flow of direction as compared to vertically is more efficient as it offers less resistance to the flow and with the use of a diagonal screen the contact surface area also increased. Diagonally screens are easy to clean. A perforated platform is provided at the top of the screen to collect the large floated waste captured by the screen. If any liquid waste is there is drops down from the perforated platform and solid waste stays on the top of the platform. The screen should be cleaned periodically so that chocking of the screen does not take place. The waste collected on the perforated platform is dumped or incineration. Figure 5.3[(a) and (b)] shows the section and plan of the coarse screen with the placement of the screen and perforated platform. A coarse screen is also known as a rack screen.

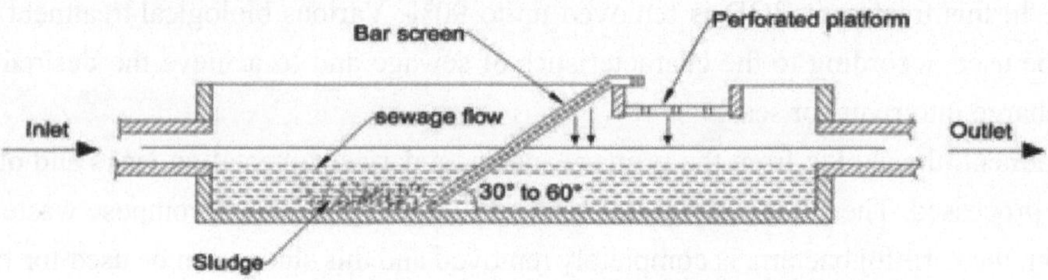

(a) Section

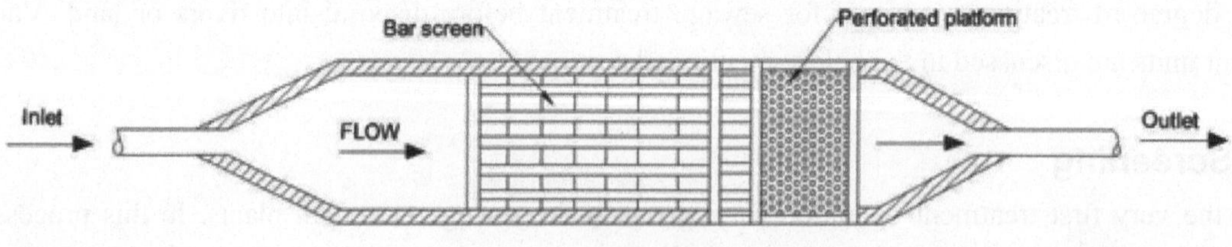

(b) Plan

Figure 5.3: Coarse screen

ii) Medium screen: In medium screen the size of the opening of the mesh is between 10 mm to 40 mm. With the help of a medium screen, some organic matter can also be removed. The material collected by the medium screen can be removed mechanically or manually. Manually cleaning is done on a small sewage treatment plant. It is done by using rakes to remove the waste from the screen.

iii) Fine screen: Fine screen are made of thin wire mesh or perforated metal sheet. The opening of perforated plate is range between 1 mm to 3 mm. This screen is very useful as compared to another size as it help in removing about 20 % of suspended particles from the sewage. There is a problem with this screen as due to the smaller size of the opening they get clogged very often and have to clean frequently. This type of screen is mostly use in treatment plants where industrial waste is treated.

5.2.3 Grit Chamber

The waste in sewage contains various inorganic impurities such as sand, stone, brick ballast, waste from glass and metal industries etc. together known as grit waste. This grit comes into sewage treatment plants from road surfaces through street inlets, service workshops, construction sites, garages, etc. During rain falls the waste from the road falls into the storm drain and reaches to the treatment plant. This grit has to be removed from sewage otherwise it will lead to the blockage of the sewage treatment line, and damage the machinery part in the treatment plant. This girt is removed from the sewage with the help of grit chamber. This grit chamber helps in removing the grit from the sewage. They are placed after screening and before the primary sedimentation tank. These tanks do not help in decomposing organic impurities. This chamber are generally rectangular in shape with their length varies from 10 to 15 m. The velocity of sewage is kept around 20 cm/sec to 35 cm/sec. The grit which is present in sewage have a relative density ranges from 2 to 5. There is a pit at the bottom of the grit chamber as shown in figure 5.4. The grit is removed from this pit hole. For controlling the velocity of sewage in grit chamber the weir are placed at the before the outlet pipe. Two grit chamber are constructed in parallel in case one is cleaning the other can be used for removing particles. The grit chamber is cleaned mechanically or manually. The waste collected from the grit chamber is disposed of by filling the low lying area near the grit chamber. The waste from grit chamber is such that it does not cause any pollution.

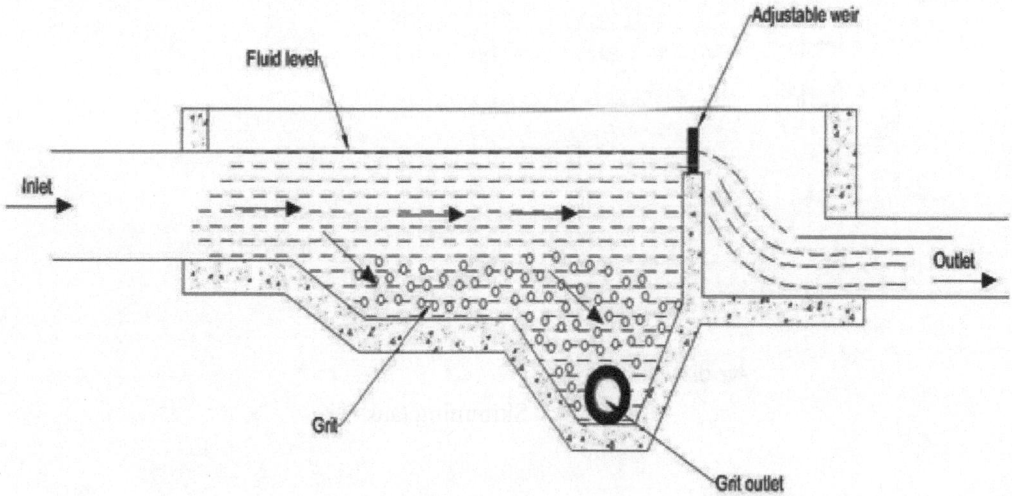

Figure 5.4: Grit Chamber

5.2.4 Skimming tank

Waste from kitchen, sanitary, garages, hospital, hotels, restaurant, butcher shops etc. contains a large quantity of grease, oil and fat. This oil, grease and fat substance is having density lighter than water so they float on the surface of the sewage waste and form scum layer on the surface. Due to this scum layer the diffusion of oxygen from the surface do not take place which in turn effect the decomposition of organic waste by aerobic bacteria. This scum also affect the oxidation process in sewage treatment plant.

Due to this reason it is necessary to remove the oil, grease and fat substance from the sewage waste. For the removal of grease and oil, skimming tank is installed in treatment plant.

This skimming tank has an air diffuser at the bottom of the tank which release air inside the tank as shown in figure 5.5. This air traps the grease and oil with them and brings on the surface of the tank. Skimming tank have a depth of around 1 m. At the inlet of the tank a baffle wall is constructed which help in discharging the inlet inside the tank and proper mixing of air with sewage waste can take place. Scrum trough is made at the top of the tank to collect the grease, oil and fat substance. Outlet is connected at the lower portion of the tank so that no oil substance can enter into outlet pipe. The detention time is kept around 5 minute. At the bottoms of the tank the perforated plates are installed through which diffused air enter into the tank. The waste collected from skimming tank is disposed of by burning or filling the pit. Skimming tank also helps in aeration of waste which in turns helps in flocculation of colloidal particles which can easily settle in sedimentation tank. This tank also helps in removing contaminated gases from the sewage waste.

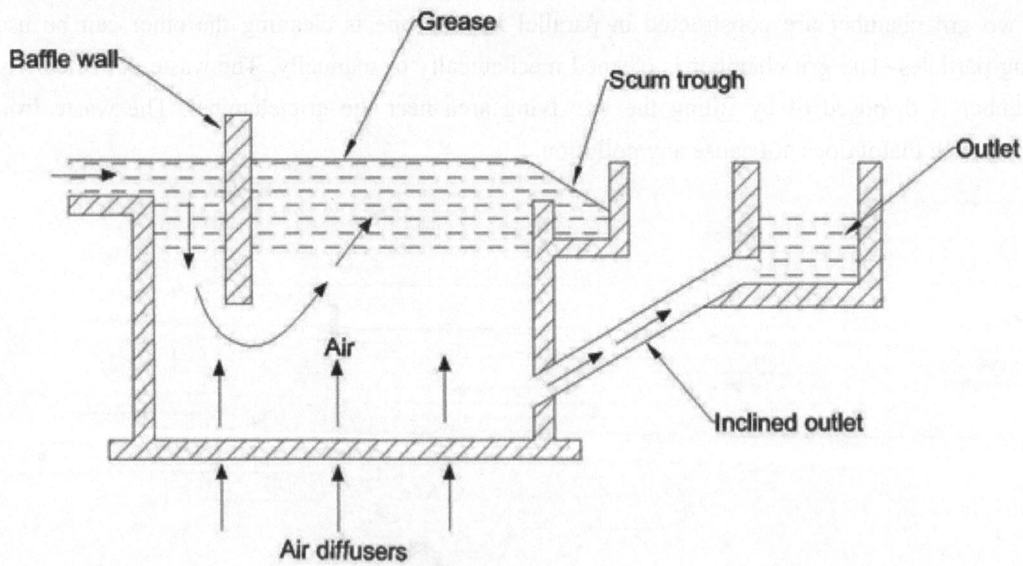

Figure 5.5: Skimming tank

5.2.5 Sedimentation of sewage

Sewage after passing through coarse screen, fine screen, skimming tank and grit chamber it still contains a large amount of fine suspended minerals and organic matter which if do not removed from sewage will create disturbance to the biological treatment units of sewage treatment plants. These impurities will blocks the pores of trickling filter and the diffused aeration system will impede which in turns effect the efficiency of activated sludge process. So it becomes very important to removes this imputes before biological treatment process. Sedimentation tank is used for removing the mineral organic matter by help of gravitational forces and this matter settles at the bottom of the tank.

Sedimentation of sewage is done by two methods:

I. Plain sedimentation

II. Sedimentation using coagulants

Sedimentation tanks can be classified based on the shape and size of the tanks. They are:

1. **Rectangular sedimentation tank:** As the name suggested these tanks are rectangular in shape having length varies from 20 m to 55 m and their width varies from 10 m to 15 m. depth of these tanks ranges from 2.5 m to 3.5 m. Flow velocity of sewage is kept around 30 cm/minute to 60 cm/minute. Detention time for the sewage is kept between 1 hour to 3 hour. If we increase the detention time for the sedimentation tanks then organic matter present in the sewage creates septic state in the sedimentation tank. Horizontal flow occur in these tanks. An inlet channel and outlet channel are present at each ends of the tank as shown in figure 5.6. Baffle walls are provided near the inlet channel to reduce the velocity of the flow of sewage. Lesser the turbulent in the sedimentation tank result in the better settlement of the mineral impurities. The bottom of the sedimentation tank has a slope against the flow direction. This is done so that the sludge do not comes out along the flow. This sludge is removed periodically from the bottom of the tank through sludge pipe as shown in figure 5.6.

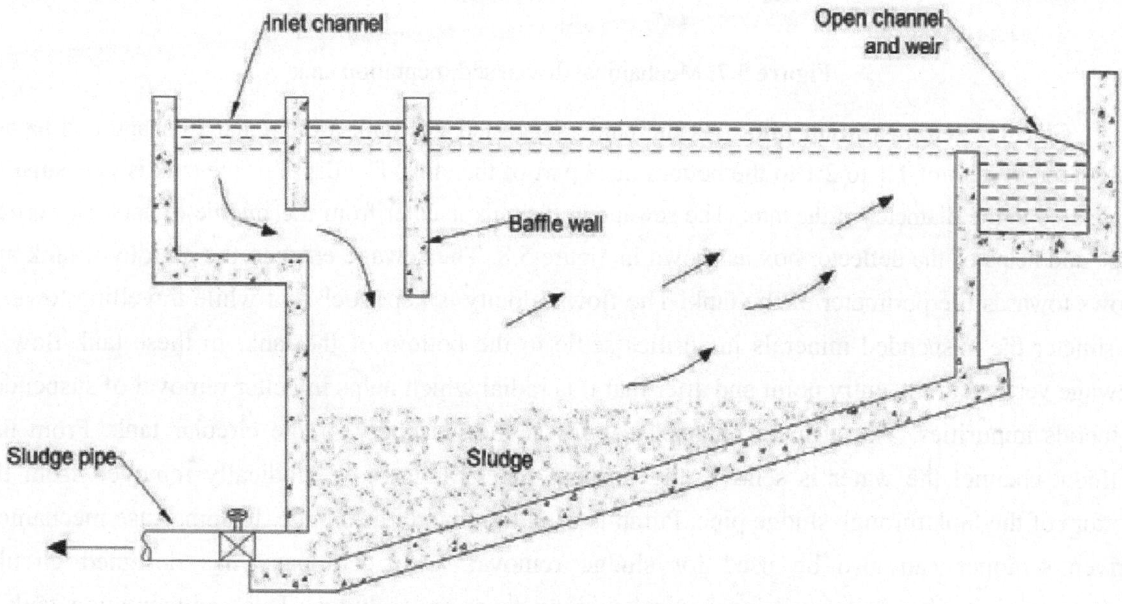

Figure 5.6: Rectangular sedimentation tank

Sludge removal is done by mechanical method. In these method scraper are used to remove the sludge from the bottom of the tank. Motor is used to continuously movement of scraper. This scraper put the removed sludge into sludge pit. Sludge from sludge pit is pumped out using pump and from there it is send to the sludge digester for further treatment. The scum which is present on the top surface of the water is also removed by scraper. Figure 5.7 shows the mechanical method for sludge removal from sedimentation tank. The sludge has to be removed periodically from the tank otherwise anaerobic digestion in the tank starts and generation of foul gases start which indirect affect the sedimentation process.

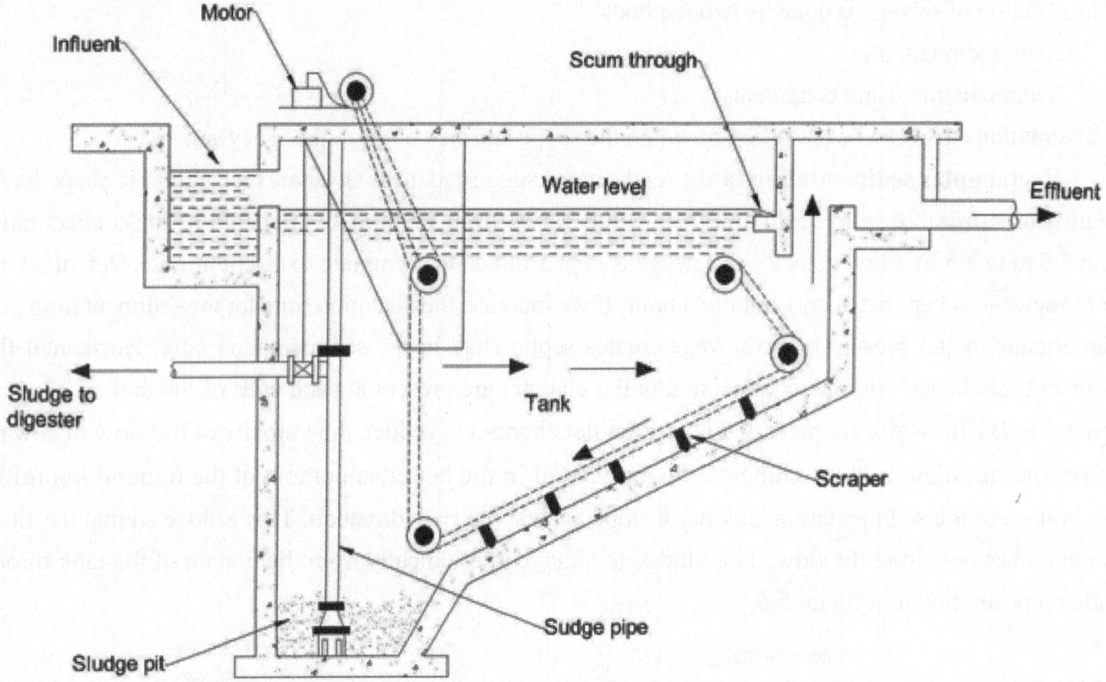

Figure 5.7: Mechanical driven sedimentation tank

2. **Circular sedimentation tank:** As the name suggested this tank are circular in shape and having side slope in ratio of 1:1 to 2:1 to the bottom most part of the tank. The depth of the tank is very small as compared to the diameter of the tank. The sewage in the tank is enter from the middle of tank by vertical pipe and helps of the deflector box as shown in figure 5.8. The sewage enter to the middle of tank and flows towards the perimeter of the tank. The flow velocity is kept such that while travelling towards perimeter the suspended minerals impurities settle to the bottom of the tank. In these tank flow of sewage vertical at the entry point and after that it is radial which helps in better removal of suspended minerals impurities. The effluent channel is built at the periphery of the circular tank. From this effluent channel the water is send to the effluent pipe. Sludge is periodically removed from the bottom of the tank through sludge pipe. Pump is used to remove the sludge. In some case mechanical driven scrapper can also be used for sludge removal. Door Company has designed circular sedimentation tank which used mechanical method to remove sludge. This sedimentation tank is operated with coagulation and known as Dorr-clarifier.

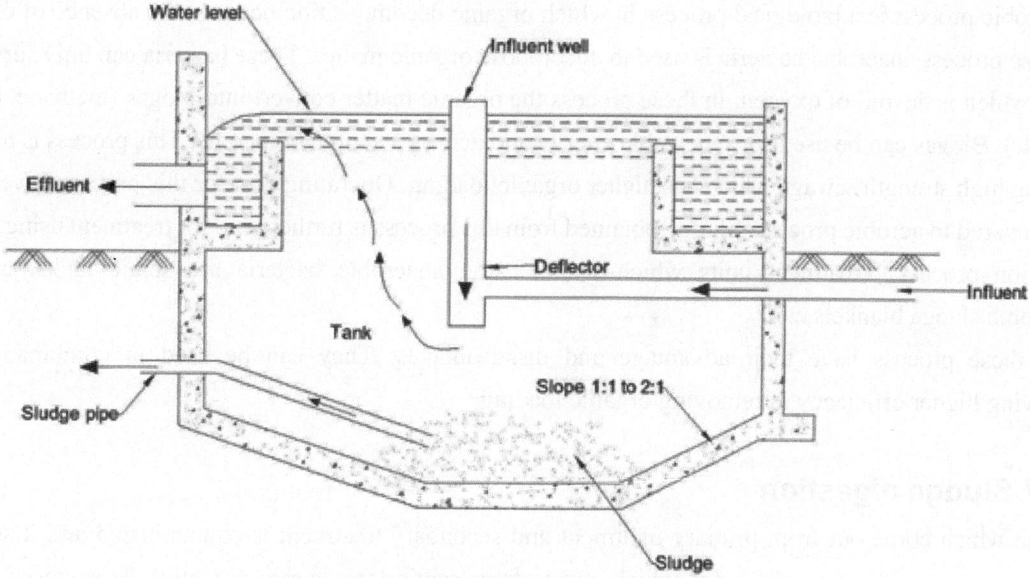

Figure 5.8: Circular sedimentation tank

3. Hopper bottom sedimentation tank: These tank have inverted cone shaped bottom and rectangular shape from the top surface. Hopper are made along the flow of direction at the bottom of the tank. In these method the sedimentation of suspended minerals impurities done more effectively and sludge collected at the hopper bottom. Flow of the sewage is horizontal and baffles wall is provided at the entry of the inlet channel to reduce the settling velocity.

5.2.6 Aerobic and anaerobic process

For the sewage treatment, aerobic and anaerobic process are two most important treatment methods which help in reducing the organic loading from sewage. This both process occur in secondary treatment of wastewater treatment plants. Aerobic and anaerobic process both helps in removing the organic contaminants from sewage but both these process required different biological conditions for their removal process to occur.

Aerobic process is a biological treatment process in which micro-organism required oxygen to break complex organic matter into simple new organic forms and gases like carbon dioxide etc. for this process aerobic bacteria is required which in turn required oxygen for decomposition. Continuously oxygen is maintained in the treatment process by using aeration pump. This process is very efficient in removing organic matter and nutrients from sewage. There is no production of biogas from this process. These process require a lot of electricity to operate as continuous aeration has to be done. The sludge produce from these process is further send to the sludge digestion unit for decomposition. Aerobic process is generally used to treat sewage which is having low to medium strength (organic loading lower than 1000 mg/l in terms of BOD). Treatment units which works on aerobic process are activated sludge process, trickling filters, contact beds etc.

Anaerobic process is a biological process in which organic decomposition occur in the absence of oxygen. In these process anaerobic bacteria is used to decompose organic matter. These bacteria can only survive in place which is devoid of oxygen. In these process the organic matter convert into biogas (methane, carbon dioxide). Biogas can be used for renewable energy and acts as a source of income. This process is used for treating high strength sewage which has higher organic loading. Operating cost for this process is very low as compared to aerobic process. Sludge obtained from this process is further send for treatment using sludge digestion process. Treatment units which works using anaerobic bacteria are septic tanks, up-flow anaerobic sludge blankets etc.

Both these process have their advantage and disadvantages. They can be used in combination for achieving higher efficiency in removing organic loading.

5.2.7 Sludge digestion

Sludge which come out from primary treatment and secondary treatment is contaminated and it starts to decompose as the time pass. Sludge which comes from septic tank is also not fully decomposed. These sludge cannot be left as such as they are highly contaminated with bacteria. These sludge is further treated by using biological digestion and the process is known as sludge digestion. The process of sludge digestion is a very complex process and special tank has to be constructed for digestion process. In sludge digestion process the decomposition of organic matter present in sludge take place. In sludge digestion process major decomposition is done by anaerobic bacteria which converts organic matter into gases (methane, carbon mono-oxide, nitrogen etc.), supernatant liquid (this liquid contains volatile colloidal matter) and digested sludge.

5.2.7.1 Different process in sludge digestion

Three different process occur in sludge digestion. They are:

i) **Acid fermentation:** These is the first process which occur in sludge digestion. In this stage the anaerobic bacteria break down the sugar, cellulose and compound containing soluble nitrogen. Due to their breakdown the organic acids and gases formation take place. Around 15 days required for this process and there is decrease in pH of sludge to 5-6. Odour of rotten egg produced during these process. Hydrogen sulphide and carbon dioxide gases released.

ii) **Acid regression:** These is the second process to occur in sludge digestion. In these stage the decomposition of compounds contains nitrogenous and organic acids to carbonate and ammonia. These stage last for around 3 months. pH of the digested sludge increase in these stages to around 7.

iii) **Alkaline fermentation:** These is the final process to occur in sludge digestion. In these stage the matter which are more resistant to dissolve get digested. There is no smell remain in the sludge after these process. pH of sludge is above 7 in these stage. Sludge after these stage take a shape of granular. These process take about one month to complete.

About more than 150 days are in total required to complete these three process of digestion of sludge. Temperature of around 27°C is kept in these stages. Complete digestion of sludge is still carried out after these stages. About 4 more weeks is required for complete digestion. For these 4 weeks the temperature is kept 35°C.

5.2.7.2 Sludge digestion Tank

Sludge digestion tank is water proof tank constructed using reinforced cement concrete or brick masonry. This tank is constructed in such a way that 1/3rd part remain above the ground level while remaining part is below the ground level. These tank can be rectangular, circular or square in shape, but preference is given to circular tank. Diameter of circular tank ranges from 6 m to 40 m while depth varies from 3 m to 12m. Gas dome is made at the top of the tank to collected the gases as shown in figure 5.9. Tank bottom is made up of hopper bottom to collect the digested sludge. Tank volume is kept such that around 35 liters to 80 liters/person for 30 days storage. Raw sludge from primary and secondary treatment enters from top of the tank and digested sludge removes from the bottom of the tank.

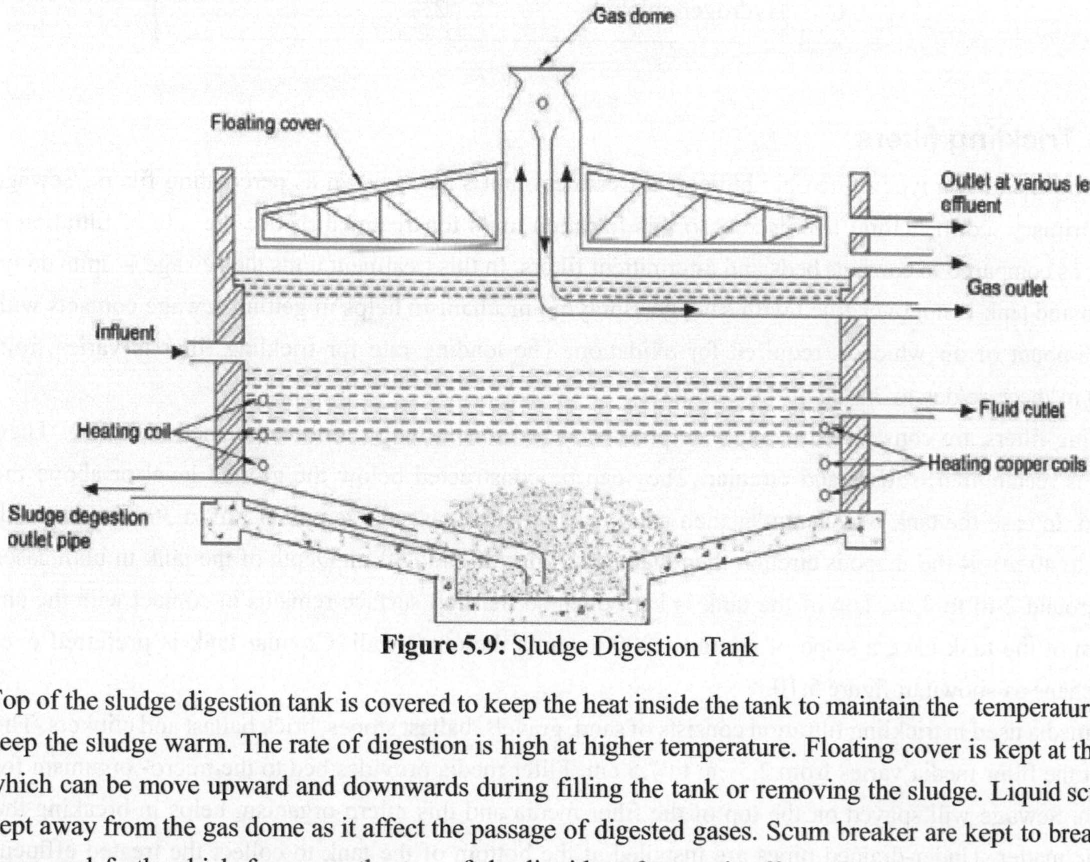

Figure 5.9: Sludge Digestion Tank

Top of the sludge digestion tank is covered to keep the heat inside the tank to maintain the temperature and keep the sludge warm. The rate of digestion is high at higher temperature. Floating cover is kept at the top which can be move upward and downwards during filling the tank or removing the sludge. Liquid scum is kept away from the gas dome as it affect the passage of digested gases. Scum breaker are kept to break the scum and forth which forms on the top of the liquid surface as it affects the digestion process. These scums are breaks by using water jets on the top of surface. Mechanical agitator are used to mix the raw sludge with digester sludge so that digestion process start early and good mixing occurred.

Heating coils are placed inside the tank to increase the temperature of the sludge as rate of digestion increase as temperature increase. Copper coils are used for heating and they are placed inside wall of the tank. Fluid outlet are made on the vertical walls to remove the supernatant liquid from the tank. Gases outlet are kept at the top to remove the gases from the gas dome. Sludge digestion tank produce around 0.028 m^3/person/day of gases. Percentage of different gases produced from sludge digestion tanks is given in table 5.2.

Table 5.2: Composition of gases released from sludge digestion tank

S. No	Name of gas	Percentage
1	Methane	60% - 70%
2	Carbon dioxide	15% - 30%
3	Nitrogen	5% - 15%
4	Hydrogen	1% - 4%
5	Carbon Mono-oxide	1%
6	Hydrogen sulphide	2%

5.2.8 Trickling filters

Trickling filters is a type of aerobic biological treatment unit's also known as percolating filters. Sewage from primary sedimentation tank is sent to this filtration units for treatment hence the rate of filtration is higher as compared to contacts beds and intermittent filters. In this treatment units the sewage is sprayed on the top and tank is not over filled with sewage. Spraying mechanism helps in getting sewage contacts with more amount of air which is required for oxidation. The loading rate for trickling filter is varies from 12000 m^3/hectare/day to 34000 m^3/hectare/day.

Trickling filters are constructed using waterproof material mixed with reinforced cement concrete. Their shape is rectangular, square and circular. They can be constructed below the ground level or above the ground. In case the tank is rectangular then its dimension varies as such length (15 m to 30 m) and width (20 m to 40 m). If the shape is circular then diameter varies 20 m to 30 m. Depth of the tank in both cases kept around 2 m to 3 m. Top of the tank is kept open so that top surface remains in contact with the air. Bottom of the tank have a slope of around 1:200 towards the outer wall. Circular tank is preferred over other shape as shown in figure 5.10.

Filter media used in trickling filtration consists of sand, gravels, ballast stones, brick ballast and clinkers. The size of the filter media varies from 2.5 cm to 7.5 cm. Filter media provides bed to the micro- organism for growth. Sewage will spayed on the top of the filter media and this micro-organism helps in breaking the organic matter. Under-drained pipes are installed at the bottom of the tank to collect the treated effluent and send to the outlet pipe.

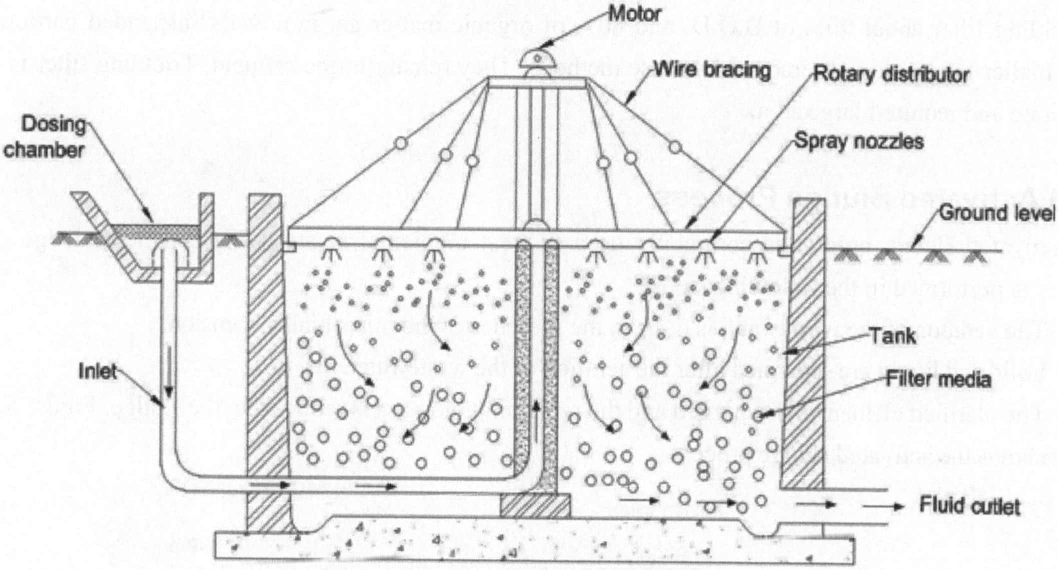

Figure 5.10: Circular trickling filter

Tricking filter specialty is that sewage is dripped or sprayed on the filter media. Special mechanical distributors are installed in the trickling filter to do spraying. They are:

a) **Fixed distributor:** In this system the distribution pipes are installed at regular intervals above the filter media. This distributors have sprayed nozzles. The sewage from primary treatment send to this distribution pipes with sufficient pressure which helps in spraying from nozzles and comes in contact with air from where it gets sufficient oxygen. Fixed distributor spraying nozzles is shown in figure 5.11.

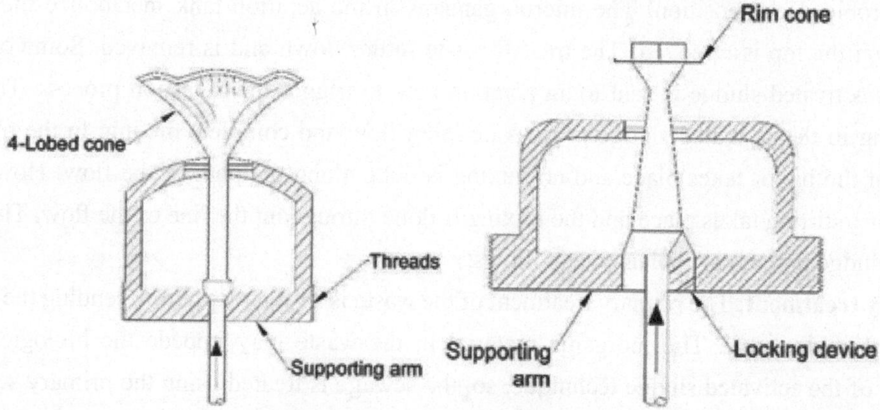

Figure 5.11: Spraying nozzles

b) **Moving distributor:** As the name suggested these distributors are continuously moving over the filter media at a slow speed. Motors are installed which help in movement of distributors. With the help of these distributors same amount of sewage get sprayed over the filter media. Now a days in trickling filter only moving distributors are used.

In trickling filter about 90% of B.O.D. and 80% of organic matter get removed. Suspended particles of very smaller in size do not removed by these methods. They remain in the effluent. Trickling filter is easy to operate and required large area.

5.2.9 Activated Sludge Process

The activated sludge process is commonly used to treat municipal wastes. The activated sludge process is performed in the following steps:

(1) The aeration of the wastewater is done in the presence of the microbial suspension.

(2) Solid and liquid are separated after the aeration of the wastewater.

(3) The clarified effluent is discharged and the remaining biomass is returned to the sludge. Figure 5.12 shows the activated sludge process.

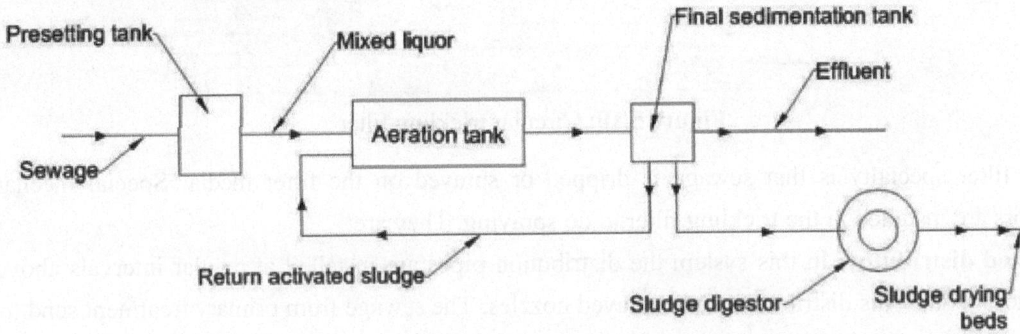

Figure 5.12: Activated sludge process

An aeration basin is used in the activated sludge process. The organic wastewater is sent to this basin and aerated for aerobic decomposition. The microorganisms in the aeration tank metabolize the waste. The scum formed on the top is removed. The treated waste settles down and is removed. Some of the sludge also known as activated sludge is sent to an aeration tank to trigger the digestion process. There are two types of mixing in the activated sludge process i.e. plug flow and complete mixing. In the plug flow, an orderly flow of the liquor takes place and no mixing is done along the path of the flow. However, in the complete mixing stirring takes place and the mixing is done throughout the line of the flow. The process of the activated sludge process is explained as follows:

(1) **Primary treatment**: The primary treatment of the waste is mandatory before sending the waste to the activated sludge tank. The inorganic material in the waste may impede the biological treatment process of the activated sludge technique, so, the sewage is treated using the primary sedimentation tank and filters to remove the inorganic impurities.

(2) **Seeding:** The activated sludge from the final sedimentation tank is added to the raw sewage for the first treatment. The amount of activated sludge is taken from 25% to 40 %. The liquid mixed with the activated sludge is also known as the mixed liquor. The mixing of the activated sludge in the raw sewage is called seeding. The seeding of the sewage is very important to enhance the efficiency of the activated sludge process.

(3) **Aeration of mixed liquor**: The waste is further proceeded to the aeration tank. It is stirred and aerated in the presence of the microorganisms. Microorganisms and bacteria eat the waste and convert it into stable waste. The detention time for the aeration tank is 4 to 6 hours. The stable wastewater remains non-odorous.

(4) **Final sedimentation**: The flocs are formed during the aeration process. These flocs are settled down and contain fine suspended solids. The sewage is released in the sedimentation tank. The sludge that settles down is known as the activated sludge. The sludge at the bottom is sent to the sludge digester tank. Scan the QR code to learn more about the activated sludge process.

5.2.10 Disposal of Sewage

The treated sewage can be disposed of in many ways depending on the extent of the stability of the treated sewage. The different methods of disposal are listed as follows:

(1) Disposal in water channel, river or sea
(2) Application on land
(3) Incineration
(4) Filtration
(5) Drying on lagoon beds

(1) **Disposal in water channels, rivers or seas:** The partially treated sewage can be disposed of in the river or water channel. The depth at the point of disposal should be sufficient for the disposal of the waste. The direction of the wind current is also determined before the disposal of the sewage. It helps avoid the foul smell of sewage in the cities.

(2) **Application on land:** The treated sewage can be used for agricultural purposes. The sludge is spread in the fields and plowed. The sludge is buried in the trenches and covered with the soil layer. The ground is plowed after two months. The fertility of the soil is enhanced by this process.

(3) **Incineration:** Incineration is the process of disposing of the sewage by burning the sludge. The incineration technique reduces the volume of the waste by 90%. Incineration is widely used for the disposal of the waste. The driers are used to dry the sewage and it can be incinerated in the furnaces.

(4) **Filtration:** The volume of the sludge can be reduced by removing the water from it. The process of reduction of volume of the sludge by removal of the water is known as filtration. The press filter, vacuum filter, or heat drying can be used for filtration.

(5) **Drying on lagoon beds:** The lagoons are shallow pits. The depth of the lagoons is around 1.5 m. The bottom of the lagoons up to 30 cm is filled with pebbles, ash, clinkers, etc. Sludge in the lagoons is filled and left for 2 to 6 months. The lime powder can be used for removal of the odour. It can be spread over the waste.

5.2.11 Oxidation Ditch

The oxidation ditches are the improved form of the activated sludge process. The oxidation ditches are capable of complete biological treatment at low costs. The oxidation ditches are preferred for the small towns. The oxidation ditch is a shallow and oval type of ditch. The details and construction of the oxidation ditch are explained as follows:

(1) **Shape:** The oxidation ditch is of oval-shaped and shallow in depth. The ditch is fitted with a cylindrical cage.

(2) **Size of the oxidation ditch:** The length of the ditch varies from 200 m to 1000 m. The width varies from 1 m to 5 m while the depth is taken from 1 m to 1.5 m. The diameter of the cylindrical cage is 75 cm.

(3) **Motor:** A motor is fitted in the cylindrical cage which can move at 75 rpm speed. It helps in the aeration of the sewage. Figure 5.13 shows the oxidation ditch.

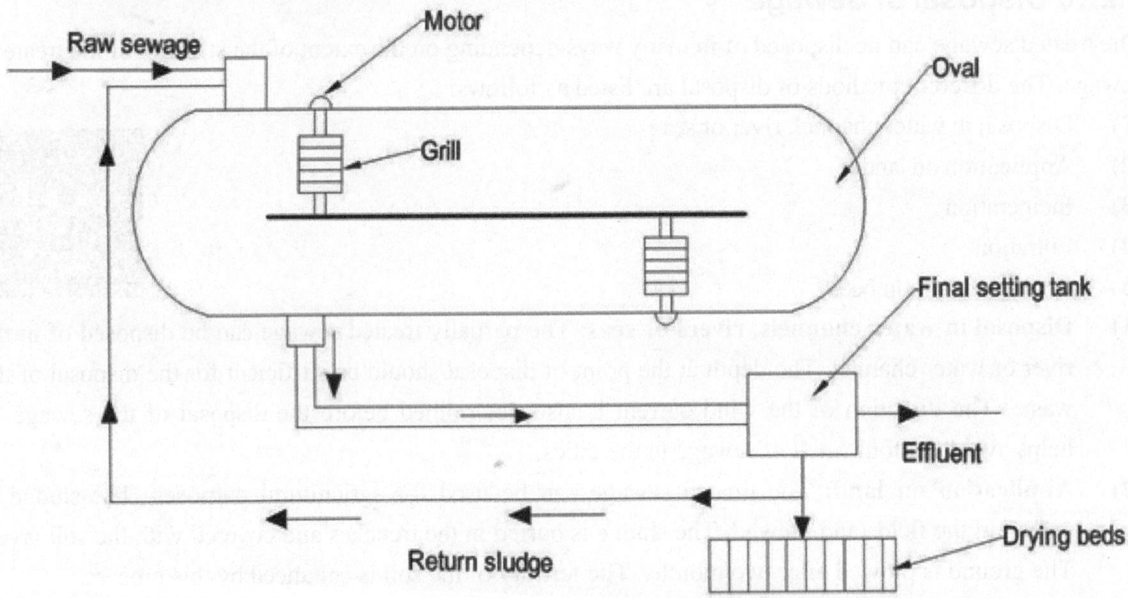

Figure 5.13: Oxidation ditch

The sewage is fed to the aeration cylinder that rotates the sewage. An aerobic process decomposes the sewage. The clean flow is achieved by the amount of sewage fed to the unit and the aeration of the ditch. The treated sewage is supplied to the sedimentation tank for further processing. The detention period of the oxidation ditch is 10 to 15 hours. The oxidation ditch can remove up to 95% of the total suspended solids while 98% to 99% of the BOD can be achieved.

5.2.12 OXIDATION POND

The oxidation ponds are also known as sewage lagoons or oxidation stabilization ponds. The raw sewage is kept in the oxidation pond for a long time, which replenishes the BOD and reduces the odor of the sewage. The aerobic bacteria and algae act together for the treatment of the raw sewage. The aerobic bacteria and algae work together to help each other in treating the raw sewage. The aerobic bacteria take the oxygen from the atmosphere and decompose the sewage to convert it into gases. The algae grow in the pond and consume the minerals. It spreads through the pond and produces oxygen through photosynthesis which triggers the decomposition process of the waste. The performance of the oxidation pond depends on photosynthesis, sunlight, temperature, etc. The oxidation ponds can meet 99% of the BOD while they can remove up to 96% of the suspended solids. Figure 5.14 shows the operations of the oxidation pond.

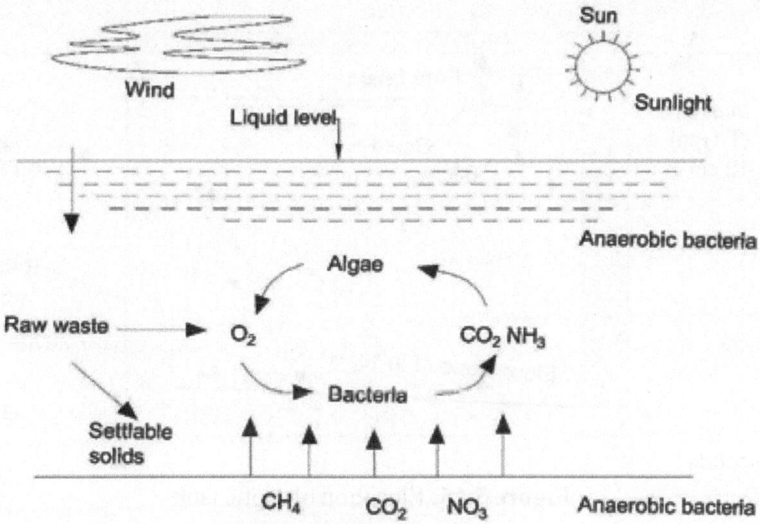

Figure 5.14: Oxidation pond

The construction of the oxidation ponds is explained as follows

(1) The oxidation pond is constructed on an embankment having sufficient size for the inspection of the tank.

(2) The depth of the tank is kept from 75 cm to 150 cm. The shallow depth of the oxidation tank helps sunlight in reaching the bottom. The length to width ration is taken 2:1.

(3) The detention period for the oxidation tanks varies from 5 days to 15 days.

(4) The oxidation ponds don't give foul smell. So, these can be constructed near the cities. The distance of such ponds can be kept 300 m from the cities.

(5) Sodium nitrate can be used for accelerating the growth of the algae.

(6) A 120 cm deep pond should be cleaned once in 6 years while a pond with 150 cm depth requires cleaning once in 12 years.

(7) Mosquito breeding will take place in the oxidation ponds. However, no chemical should be used to prevent mosquito breeding as it may destroy the algae.

5.2.13 Septic Tank

A septic tank may be defined as an underground airtight tank that receives partially treated or untreated domestic waste. The waste is treated under anaerobic conditions. The heavy solids sit at the bottom of the septic tank while the liquid and light wastes float. The septic tank is a kind of plain sedimentation tank, however, the digestion in the septic tank takes place in an anaerobic environment. Figure 5.15 shows the elevation of septic tank.

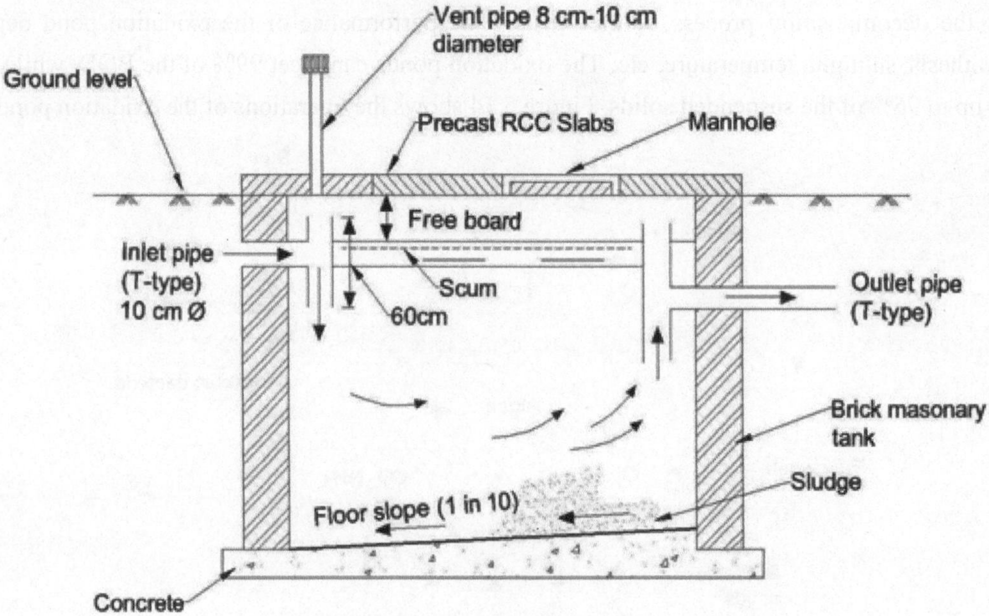

Figure 5.15: Elevation of septic tank

5.2.13.1 Features of a Septic Tank

The sewage is treated during the detention time and disposed of in the soak pit. A cover is provided in the septic tank to prevent the foul smells. The following aspects are considered while constructing a septic tank:

(1) The septic tank is constructed using the anti-corrosive material. As discussed earlier, the anaerobic conditions exist in the septic tank. So, the septic tank should be air-tight to avoid the foul smells and corrosion,

(2) There should not be currents between the outlet and the inlet. A baffle wall is constructed in the septic tank to avoid these currents.

(3) The vent pipes are provided for the ventilation purposes.

(4) Inspection of the septic tank is needed. So, a manhole is provided for periodic inspection of the tank.

(5) The top cover of the septic tank is constructed using reinforced cement concrete.

(6) The sludge should not accumulate at the bottom of the tank and should be removed periodically. The sludge can be removed manually or mechanically. In some septic tanks, the sludge removal pipe is also provided. The sludge is removed in a time interval of 6 months to 1 year.

(7) The effluent from the septic tank should not be disposed of directly into the water channels. Its disposal should be considered carefully. Figure 5.16 shows the plan of a septic tank.

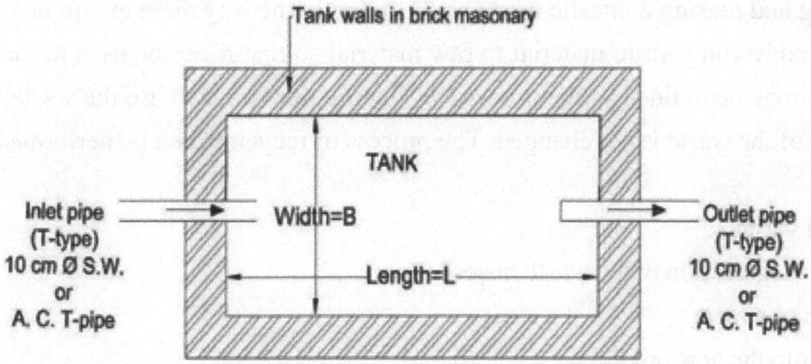

Figure 5.16: Plan of a septic tank

5.2.13.2 Design Aspects

The design and size of the septic tank depend on the number of persons who will be using the septic tank. The different design aspects of the septic tank are discussed as follows:

(1) **Tank capacity:** The capacity of the tank is designed according to the number of users. The suitable size of the septic tank for the residential colonies are given in the Table 5.3. Indian standard code IS: 2470 Part-I provides the details of suitable sizes of the septic tanks to be constructed for different types of buildings.

Table 5.3: Suitable sizes of septic tanks for residential colonies

No of users	*Length*	*Breadth*	*Liquid depth*	
			1-year cleaning interval	*2-year cleaning interval*
50	5.0 m	1.6 m	1.3 m	1.4 m
100	5.7 m	2.1 m	1.4 m	1.7 m
150	7.7 m	2.4 m	1.4 m	1.7 m
200	8.9 m	2.7 m	1.4 m	1.7 m

(2) **Shape and dimensions:** The shape of the septic tank is rectangular in most of the cases. It consists of two or three chambers. The length of the septic tank varies from 2 to 4 times of the depth of the tank. The depth is taken from 1 m to 2m.

(3) **Free board:** A freeboard of 300 mm to 500 mm is provided. The liquid capacity of the tank is taken from 90 to 115 liters per person.

(4) **Pipes:** The vent pipe of 5 cm to 10 cm diameter is taken. The diameter of the inlet and outlet pipe of 10 cm to 15 cm.

5.3 Recycling and Reuse of Domestic Waste

The domestic waste from the kitchen and houses can be recycled and reused. It will help reduce the adverse impacts of the waste on the environment and will lead to economical waste management solutions.

The terms recycling and reusing domestic waste are different in the way these are implemented. Recycling may be defined as converting waste material to raw material so that it can be used to make new products. The reuse of waste may be defined as the process of finding new ways to use the waste. In the reusing of the waste, the form of the waste is not changed. The process of recycling can be performed in the following steps:

(1) Collection of waste

(2) Separation or segregation of the waste material

(3) Cleaning and treatment

(4) Conversion into the new products

(1) Waste collection: Domestic solid waste is collected using waste collection vehicles. The government-owned vehicles collect the domestic waste door to door. The residents collect the waste in the dustbins, which are then handed over to the waste collection vehicles.

(2) Separation and segregation of the waste material: Two separate dustbins are used for wet and dry waste in the residential area. The dry waste and wet waste are collected separately in the collection vehicles too. Using some color coding on the dustbins is a general practice for this purpose. In India, the green dustbin is used for collecting the wet waste while the blue- colored dustbin is used for collecting the dry waste. The wet wastes include all the organic material coming out as domestic waste like food waste, papers, etc. The dry and wet waste is further segregated and collected in three categories at the collection center. The dry waste including plastic bottles, papers, glass, etc. are separated. The organic waste including the waste food items, leftover fruits, vegetables, etc. is separated. Domestic hazardous wastes like diapers, napkins, mosquito repellents, etc. are separated too.

(3) Cleaning and treatment: The segregated waste material is cleaned and treated for further processing. The hazardous waste is treated and disposed of in the water, land, or ocean based on the standard norms. The organic waste is collected and sent for aerobic or anaerobic treatment. The plastic waste, glass waste, metal waste, etc. are segregated and sent for cleaning so that these can be used for recycling.

(4) Conversion into the new products: The segregated waste material used for making the new products. The plastic can be melted and reformed into toys, mugs, buckets, and other useful products. The metals can be converted into utensils and other mechanical parts. The organic material is converted into compost and used for agricultural work.

The waste material can be reused without converting it into new products. The broken boxes or waste plastic buckets can be used as dustbins. The wastewater from the kitchen is used for irrigation. The waste organic matter can also be used as food for fish. The researchers have used domestic waste to grow micro algae which can be used for the production of ethanol. Ethanol has a significant economic value in the current industrial scenario.

UNIT SUMMARY

- Analysis of sewage is to be done to know about the sewage characteristics.
- Physical, chemical and biological characteristics of sewage gives the idea of organic and inorganic matter concentration.
- BOD and COD gives the idea about organic matter in sewage.
- Sewage discharge norms as per CPCB is given.
- Screening is provide in sewage treatment plant to removes large floating debris.
- A grit chamber is constructed to remove inorganic impurities from sewage.
- Skimming tank helps in removing grease, fat and oil from sewage.
- Sedimentation tank is provided to remove the suspended organic matter from sewage.
- There are two types of bacteria that help in decomposition of organic matter.
- Aerobic process occur in presence of oxygen.
- Anaerobic process occur in absence of oxygen.
- Sludge digestion is used to decompose sludge from primary treatment and secondary treatment.
- Trickling filter is an aerobic process in which sewage is treated and filter media is used.
- Activated sludge process is also an aerobic process in which activated sludge is remix which primary treated sewage so that decomposition of organic matter start early.
- After sewage is treated its effluent is discharge into river or can be used in farming.
- Oxidation pond is a technique in which aerobic, anaerobic and facultative bacteria involved for sewage treatment.
- Domestic sewage is used in fishing and irrigation purpose.
- An aeration basin is used in the activated sludge process. The organic wastewater is sent to this basin and aerated for aerobic decomposition.
- The microorganisms in the aeration tank metabolize the waste.
- The direction of the wind current is also determined before the disposal of the sewage. It helps avoid the foul smell of sewage in the cities.
- The oxidation ditches are the improved form of the activated sludge process. The oxidation ditches are capable of complete biological treatment at low costs.
- The oxidation ponds are also known as sewage lagoons or oxidation stabilization ponds.
- The raw sewage is kept in the oxidation pond for a long time, which replenishes the BOD and reduces the odor of the sewage.
- A septic tank may be defined as an underground airtight tank that receives partially treated or untreated domestic waste.
- Recycling may be defined as converting waste material to raw material so that it can be used to make new products.

EXERCISES

Multiple Choice Questions

1. What is an average amount of solids in 100 kg of sewage?
   (a) 450gm (b) 500gm
   (c) 400gm (d) 600gm
2. What should be the BOD_5 for weak strength sewage?
   (a) 350mg/l (b) 250mg/l
   (c) 500mg/l (d) All of the above
3. What should be the temperature of COD digester?
   (a) 100°C (b) 120°C
   (c) 150°C (d) None
4. What should be the opening size of coarse screens?
   (a) >50mm (b) <50mm
   (c) All of the above (d) None
5. Which of the following is an anaerobic process?
   (a) Trickling filter (b) Activated sludge Process
   (c) Septic Tank (d) None of these
6. Percentage of methane gas produced in sludge digestion tank?
   (a) 60-70 (b) 40-50
   (c) >80 (d) None of these
7. Physical characteristics of sewage has following parameters?
   (a) Turbidity (b) Solids
   (c) Chloride (d) BOD
8. Free board in the septic tank is kept:
   (a) 10 cm to 20 cm (b) 30 cm to 50 cm
   (c) 40 cm to 60 cm (d) None of the above
9. The oxidation pond can remove the suspended solid:
   (a) 99% (b) 98%
   (c) 96% (d) None of the above
10. The detention period of oxidation ditch is:
    (a) 10 to 15 hours (b) 15 to 20 hours
    (c) One day (d) None of the above

Answers of Multiple Choice Questions

1. (a), 2. (b), 3. (c), 4. (a), 5. (c), 6. (a), 7. (a), 8. (b), 9. (c), 10. (a)

Short and Long Answer Type Questions

1. Explain the primary treatment and secondary treatment in sewage
2. Write a short note on physical characteristics of sewage.
3. Enlist the conditions in which septic tank is provided.
4. What type of screen can be provided for the sewage treatment? Discuss in detail.
5. Explain the grit chamber and skimming tank
6. Explain different types of tanks used in sedimentation.
7. What do you understand by aerobic and anaerobic process?
8. What are the objects of sewage treatment?
9. Explain the septic tank with diagram.
10. Draw a neat sketch of sludge digester tank. Identify its various parts.
11. Explain the different nozzle disturbers in sludge digestion tank.
12. Explain BOD and COD.
13. Describe working of trickling filter.
14. Explain oxidation ditch and oxidation pond?
15. Explain different method of sewage disposal?
16. Explain recycling and reuse of sewage.
17. Explain the design features of a septic tank.
18. Enlist five differences in oxidation ditch and oxidation pond.
19. Explain the concept of recycling and reusing.
20. Explain the concept of activated sludge process with neat sketch.

REFERENCES AND SUGGESTED READINGS

1. Garg, S.K., Environmental Engineering Vol. I and Vol. II, Khanna Publishers
2. Sharma S.C, Environmental Engineering, Khanna Publishing House, New Delhi
3. Punmia, B C, Environmental Engineering, vol. I and II, Laxmi Publishers
4. Basak N N, Environmental Engineering, McGraw Hill Publishers.
5. Manual on water supply and treatment system, Government of India (2023)
6. Environmental (protection) act, 1986 (2016), MOEFCC, Government of India.
7. IS Code 2470, Part I
8. Bardsley DA. B. coli as an Index of Faecal Pollution of Water Supplies. J Hyg (Lond). 1926 Feb;25(1):11-25. doi: 10.1017/s0022172400017186.

REFERENCES FOR FURTHER LEARNING

1. Garg, S. K. *Water Supply Engineering*, 37st Edition Khanna publishers, New Delhi
2. Peavy, H. S., Rowe, D. R. & Tchobanoglous, G. *Environmental Engineering*, 1st Edition McGraw Hill Education, New Delhi
3. Masters, G. M & Pela, W. *Introduction to Environmental Engineering and Science*, 3[rt] Edition, Pearson Education India, Chennai
4. IS 10500:2012, *Indian Standard, Drinking water-Specification,* Bureau of Indian Standards (BIS), New Delhi
5. Government of India, *Central Pollution Control Board*, Guidelines for reuse of treated sewage in reference to item of circular economy, 2019, , CPCB, New Delhi,
6. Government of India, *Ministry of urban development*, A hand book on recent trends in technologies in sewerage system, 2012, , MOHUA, New Delhi.

CO AND PO ATTAINMENT TABLE

Course outcomes (COs) for this course can be mapped with the program outcomes (POs) after the completion of the course and a correlation can be made for the attainment of POs to analyze the gap. After proper analysis of the gap in the attainment of POs necessary measures can be taken to overcome the gaps.

Table for CO and PO attainment

Course Outcomes	Attainment of Programme Outcomes *(1- Weak Correlation; 2- Medium correlation; 3- Strong Correlation)*						
	PO-1	PO-2	PO-3	PO-4	PO-5	PO-6	PO-7
CO-1							
CO-2							
CO-3							
CO-4							
CO-5							

The data filled in the above table can be used for gap analysis.

INDEX